HIGH CHOLESTEROL

Skyhorse Publishing books may be purchased in bulk at special discounts for sales promotion, corporate gifts, fund-raising, or educational purposes. Special editions can also be created to specifications. For details, contact the Special Sales Department, Skyhorse Publishing, 555 Eighth Avenue, Suite 903, New York, NY 10018 or info@skyhorsepublishing.com.

www.skyhorsepublishing.com

10 9 8 7 6 5 4 3 2 1

Library of Congress Cataloging-in-Publication Data

Kingham, Karen.
 Eat well live well with high cholesterol : low-cholesterol recipes and tips / Karen Kingham.
    p. cm.
 Includes index.
 ISBN 978-1-60239-674-6
 1. Low-cholesterol diet--Recipes 2. Self-care, Health. I. Title.
 RM237.75.K54 2009
 641.5'63847--dc22
                            2009015873

Printed in China

IMPORTANT: Those who might be at risk from the effects of salmonella poisoning (the elderly, pregnant women, young children and those suffering from immune deficiency diseases) should consult their doctor with any concerns about eating raw eggs.

CONVERSION GUIDE: You may find cooking times vary depending on the oven you are using. For convection ovens, as a general rule, set the oven temperature to 35°F lower than indicated in the recipe.

EATWELLLIVEWELL
with HIGH
CHOLESTEROL
Low-cholesterol recipes and tips

Introductory text by Karen Kingham (nutritionist)

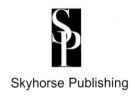

Skyhorse Publishing

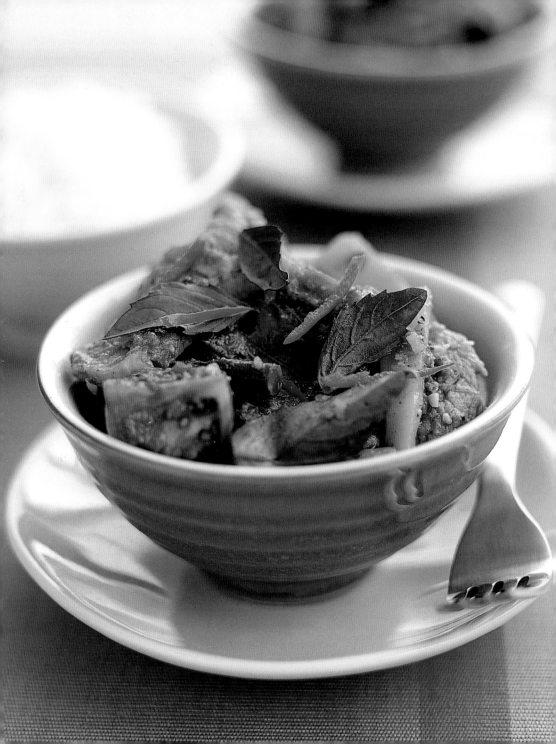

CONTENTS

LOWER CHOLESTEROL THE HEALTHY WAY

High blood cholesterol is one of the major risk factors for heart disease, which can lead to heart attack or stroke. Simply put, the higher the cholesterol level, the greater the risk. Best estimates rank cardiovascular disease (CVD) as the leading cause of death in the Western world. The expectation is that CVD will become an even greater health problem, along with obesity and diabetes, by the end of the next decade.

The good news in all of this is the lower you get your blood cholesterol, the lower your risk of CVD and the less chance you have of becoming a health statistic.

There is plenty you can do to achieve a lower blood cholesterol level, the most important being improving your diet and lifestyle. Diets to lower cholesterol have come a long way in the last 20 years. Bland high-fiber meals devoid of fat are out, flavorsome and colorful meals using the right fats are in. So take the opportunity to change your life—enjoy the recipes in this book with family and friends, lower your cholesterol and live a longer healthier life.

What is cholesterol?

Cholesterol is a waxy, fatty substance made naturally, in amounts determined by your genetic make-up, by the liver. We all need a certain amount of cholesterol to make hormones, coat our nerve cells so signals travel properly, and form the outer membranes of our body's cells. Cholesterol is not bad for us when we have it in the right amounts.

Our body also gets small amounts of cholesterol from the foods we eat, such as shellfish, meat, chicken, eggs, butter, cheese and whole milk. Foods with saturated and trans fats can upset the body's cholesterol balance by causing your liver to make more cholesterol than it otherwise would.

Because cholesterol is a fat and can't dissolve in the blood, it must get to and from the cells via transporters or carriers known as lipoproteins, of which there are two types.

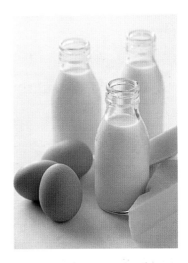

Low-density lipoprotein or LDL cholesterol: This is found in the greatest amounts and is the one you most need to worry about.

LDL's main job is to take cholesterol from the liver to the body cells where it is needed. Too much LDL causes a build-up of cholesterol on the inside of blood vessel walls which is not good for your health.

High-density lipoprotein or HDL cholesterol: This is the cholesterol you want to have more of. HDL tidies up excess cholesterol, picking it up from your blood vessels and taking it back to your liver.

The trouble with too much LDL cholesterol

Too much LDL cholesterol in your blood causes the excess to be deposited in the blood vessels. Over time, the cholesterol, along with other substances, builds up in the vessel walls, causing them to narrow and then harden—think of the sludge you might get clogging up your drain pipes at home. This process is known as atherosclerosis.

Cholesterol deposited in the blood vessels is also more susceptible to a process known as oxidation. When LDL is oxidized, it becomes more irritating to the blood vessel, causing inflammation, which then accelerates the process of atherosclerosis.

Depending on your genes, diet and lifestyle, atherosclerosis can start as early as childhood and can become quite advanced by the time you reach middle age.

Atherosclerosis is involved in the progression of a number of diseases:

- **Coronary heart disease** occurs when the blood vessels to the heart are affected by atherosclerosis and can lead to angina (chest pain) or a heart attack.
- **Cerebrovascular disease** is caused by narrowing or blockages in blood vessels to the brain and can result in a stroke.
- **Peripheral vascular disease** is the result of narrowing or blockage of the blood

7

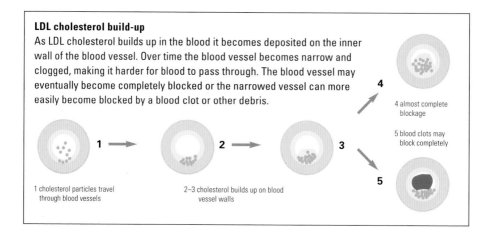

LDL cholesterol build-up

As LDL cholesterol builds up in the blood it becomes deposited on the inner wall of the blood vessel. Over time the blood vessel becomes narrow and clogged, making it harder for blood to pass through. The blood vessel may eventually become completely blocked or the narrowed vessel can more easily become blocked by a blood clot or other debris.

4 almost complete blockage

5 blood clots may block completely

1 cholesterol particles travel through blood vessels

2–3 cholesterol builds up on blood vessel walls

vessels in parts of the body other than the brain or heart, such as the legs, arms, stomach, kidneys or other organs.

These diseases of the heart and blood vessels caused by atherosclerosis are collectively known as CVD, the number one cause of death for men and women in Western countries.

Your cholesterol target

If your blood cholesterol is high, your doctor will give you advice on the best level for which to aim. Regardless of how high your blood cholesterol is, the lower you get your LDL cholesterol, the better off you'll be.

The American Heart Association recommends you keep blood cholesterol levels in the following range*:

Total cholesterol	less than 200 mg/dL
LDL cholesterol	less than 100 mg/dL
HDL cholesterol	more than 60 mg/dL

*Depending upon where in the world you live these may differ.

What affects cholesterol levels?

In the Western world, there are a number of factors that may cause your cholesterol to rise. Some of these you can change, some you can't.

These are the factors you can't change

- **Your age and gender:** Blood cholesterol tends to rise as we get older and is usually higher in men than women, until after menopause. A woman's cholesterol may quickly catch up to that of men of a similar age after menopause.
- **Your inheritance:** High blood cholesterol can run in families and your genes may put you at greater risk.

> **How common is high cholesterol?**
> Thirty to fifty per cent of adults in Western countries have high blood cholesterol. Despite knowing about the harmful effects of high cholesterol and understanding how easy it can be to lower it, the numbers of people with high blood cholesterol has changed little in some countries since the 1980s.

These are the factors you can change

- **Your weight:** The world's population has become dramatically heavier over the past 20 years. Rates of overweight and obesity in Western nations have climbed to as much as 60 percent. And as our weight increases, so too is the likelihood that LDL cholesterol will be higher and HDL will be lower than is ideal.
- **Your diet:** Eating a diet high in saturated fat is one of the most significant causes of high LDL cholesterol. Major sources of saturated fat in our diet include butter, cream, cheese and other full-fat dairy products, the fat associated with meat and poultry (especially from skin), sausages, salami and other processed meats. Significant amounts are also found in many baked goods (cookies, cakes, pies, pastries), fried takeout foods and snack foods (chocolate, potato chips, corn chips and cheese-flavored snacks).
- **How much you move:** Being more physically active will not only lower your LDL cholesterol but improve your risk-factor profile for CVD by lowering blood pressure, reducing insulin resistance, helping with weight control and improving mental health. Being more physically active will also lower your risk of developing type 2 diabetes, osteoporosis, obesity, breast and colon cancer, and depression.

What about triglycerides?

If you've had a cholesterol test, it is likely that the results included information about triglycerides: these are a type of fat found in your blood. Triglycerides come from the fats in the food you eat and are also made in the body—especially if you eat too many calories—your body then turns them into triglycerides (fat).

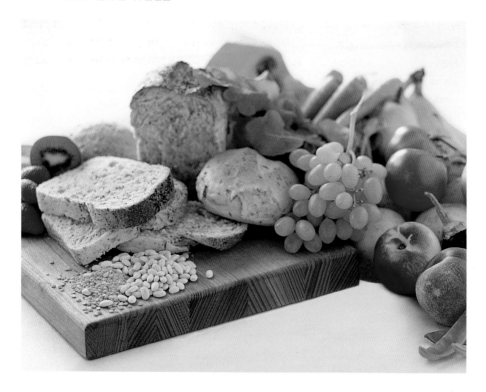

The link between high triglycerides and CVD remains uncertain, but when triglycerides are high, your risk of heart problems usually rises, especially if your LDL cholesterol is also high.

Triglyceride levels tend to be high if you smoke, drink alcohol to excess, are obese, don't exercise enough or eat too many refined carbohydrates. Type 2 diabetes and liver and kidney diseases also increase your chances of having high triglycerides, as can your genes.

Ideally, you should aim to keep your triglycerides less than 150 mg/dL. Do this by following the advice given in this book, giving up smoking, drinking less alcohol and eating less refined and more whole grain and low-GI carbohydrates.

Risk factors for cardiovascular disease

If you have high blood cholesterol, have you considered how high your risk of CVD is and what your chances are of having a heart attack or stroke? These are important questions that everyone with high cholesterol should know the answers to. The most accurate answer—your risk in percentage terms—is best calculated by your doctor. However, you can get a rough idea by considering how many of these risk factors apply to you:

- High total and LDL cholesterol
- Low HDL cholesterol
- High triglycerides
- Cigarette smoking
- High blood pressure (for example, over 140/90 mmHg)
- Overweight and obesity
- Inactivity
- Diabetes or pre-diabetes
- Stress, depression and social isolation
- Over 45 years of age
- Family history of heart disease (parent or sibling affected at less than 60 years of age)
- Kidney transplant or kidney disease
- Aboriginal or Torres Strait Islander descent
- Maori or Pacific Islander descent
- Asian or from the Indian subcontinent
- African or Mexican American

In general, the higher your LDL cholesterol level and the more risk factors you have, the greater your chances of developing CVD and having a heart attack or stroke. Fortunately, by living a healthier life you can make a real difference to many of your risk factors. In short, give up smoking, take charge of your diet and get out of the house and move more.

The issue of weight

Being overweight increases your risk of high cholesterol and CVD as well as many other health problems. Overweight is defined as having a body mass index (BMI) of 25 or more. If you know your weight and height you can work out your BMI:

$$BMI = 703 \times \frac{\text{Weight (1 lb)}}{\text{Height}^2 \text{ (in)}^2}$$

Maintaining a healthy weight
Following is a list of all the good reasons why you should aim to keep your weight down using a heart healthy diet and regular exercise:

Heart health benefits
- Lower LDL cholesterol
- Higher HDL cholesterol
- Lower triglycerides
- Lower blood pressure
- Improve insulin resistance and control blood glucose if you have diabetes
- Reduce your risk of CVD

General health benefits
- Reduce risk of type 2 diabetes
- Lower risk of some cancers
- Improve sleep apnea
- Reduce joint pain in arthritis
- Control gout
- Lower risk of gall bladder disease
- Improve asthma
- Relieve reflux
- Improve fertility

For most people their BMI is a good indicator of body fat levels and health risks. But there are some—such as athletes and those of some ethnic groups (for example, Pacific Islanders and South-East Asians)—who are the exception.

Where on your body you store your fat makes a big difference to your CVD risk. Fat stored around your tummy (apple shapes) puts you at greater risk than fat stored on your hips and thighs (pear shapes).

Checking your waist size is easy using a tape measure at the level of your belly button. Women should aim for a waist less than 31½ in and men less than 37 in. A waist size greater than this makes you a bigger candidate for a heart attack or stroke.

Healthier eating habits to lower blood cholesterol

Better eating habits and a healthier lifestyle—which includes being more active as well as giving up smoking—are two of the biggest steps you can take to lower your blood cholesterol. This is why your doctor will usually give you a chance with these before prescribing you any medication. These changes are also the best way to avoid getting high cholesterol.

Once you have commenced your plan to lower cholesterol, don't forget to visit your doctor and keep track of your progress. Anyone with high cholesterol and at high risk of CVD should have their blood cholesterol checked every year. The benefits of the changes you will make are well proven, but there's no better motivator than to see improvements in your LDL and HDL cholesterol for yourself.

Fast food, be it takeout or made at home from highly-processed ingredients, is high in saturated fat, low in fiber and contains fewer vitamins and minerals. When eaten regularly, this sort of food slows you down and makes you more likely to suffer health problems, particularly high cholesterol.

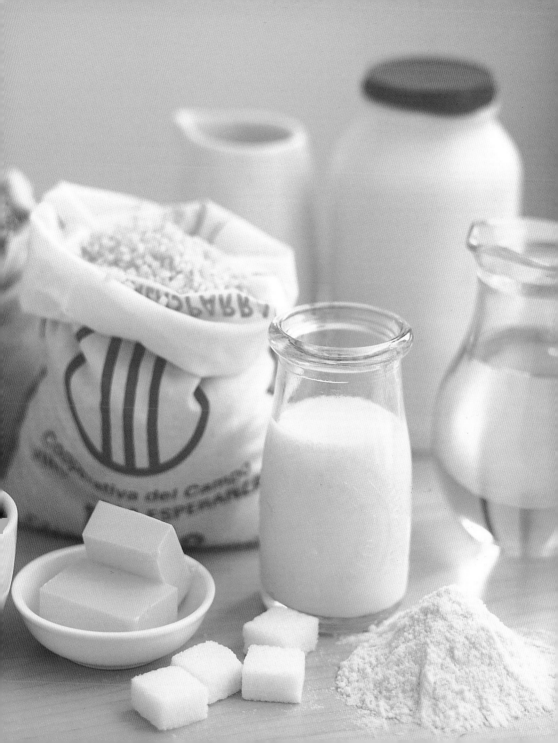

Women take special care

Cardiovascular disease claims five times the lives that breast cancer does. Yet, high blood cholesterol and CVD are often dismissed by women as being male problems. Protective female hormones give women an extra 10 to 15 years of good cardiovascular health compared to men. However, blood cholesterol levels can rise significantly after menopause. With these extra years "up your sleeve" a valuable opportunity exists to take care of yourself and intercept the consequences of menopause to live a longer, healthier life.

Advancing knowledge in nutrition tells us that while we go forward in some things, in others we go back. For the health of your heart and blood vessels going back to basics and embracing natural unprocessed foods is what you need. This doesn't mean a return to the bland, high-fiber, low-fat diets of the 1980s. Instead it means going back to more traditional foods, such as:

- whole grains, legumes and fresh fruit and vegetables for their antioxidants, phytochemicals and low-GI carbohydrates
- nuts, seeds and more fish for their healthier fats
- lean meat, chicken, seafood and low-fat dairy for vital protein.

An abundance of foods have proven heart health benefits and many will be discussed in the following pages. But no single food will keep cholesterol at bay. Success is only possible by including as many heart-friendly foods in your diet as possible. Heart healthy eating habits are additive. If you can follow all of the advice given here, there is the potential to drop blood cholesterol by as much as a 30 percent—better than some medications prescribed by your doctor.

Don't despair if you don't manage to follow all the advice given here. Start with the most important—cutting down on your saturated fat. Use our guides and tips to track down saturated fat and remove it from your diet. Once you have made this change successfully, choose another, then another, until you have made them all. If you are finding it hard to achieve our advice or if you have diabetes, kidney disease or any other serious medical problems, seek the advice of a dietitian. This will ensure your eating plan is in tune with your lifestyle and meets your individual health needs making a lower cholesterol easier to achieve.

Cut the bad fat

Just as there is good and bad blood cholesterol, there are good and bad fats. Rather than ridding your diet of all fat, the best thing you can do to get your cholesterol down is to achieve the right balance of good and bad fats.

Saturated fat is the biggest culprit for raising your LDL cholesterol level. These fats are usually of animal origin (except for palm oil and coconut fat). Trans fats come a close second in cholesterol-raising ability. Trans fats occur naturally in some foods of animal origin such as beef, lamb and dairy foods. They are also made when liquid vegetable oils are turned into hard fats (margarines and solid frying fats) for commercial food production. This process is known as hydrogenation or partial hydrogenation.

Major sources of trans fats include crackers, cookies, doughnuts, corn and potato chips, margarine, french fries and other commercially produced fried foods—anything prepared using hydrogenated or partially hydrogenated oils. Some countries have higher levels of trans fats in their foods than others, but this is changing as governments become more aware of the health threat they pose and place pressure on food industries to lower the amount of trans fats in the foods they produce. Cutting back on saturated and trans fats and using healthier monounsaturated and polyunsaturated fats will lower LDL and raise HDL cholesterol. Our easy-to-read table on the right lets you find these bad fats so you can make better choices when you shop.

Where is the bad fat?

Ridding your diet of saturated and trans fats takes time and practice. Consider the following tips for ousting these bad fellows from your life:

- Avoid butter, lard, cream, sour cream, coconut milk or cream and hard cooking margarines
- Choose lean cuts of meat and trim any remaining fat before cooking
- Choose skinless cuts of chicken or remove the skin before eating
- Eat cheese less often and choose lower fat varieties
- Avoid high-fat processed deli meats like bologna and salami
- Use low or reduced fat milks, yogurts, ice creams and custard
- Avoid deep-fried takeout foods.
- Choose tomato based pasta sauces over creamy types
- Save commercial cookies, cakes, muffins, pastries and sweets for special occasions
- Cut back on high-fat snack foods, such as chocolate bars, chips and crackers
- Cook with low-fat methods: steaming, grilling, baking and barbecuing

Make sure you include a good balance of polyunsaturated and monounsaturated fats in your diet by thinking about variety:

- Use a range of oils in your meal preparations—sunflower or canola for baking, extra virgin olive, macadamia or walnut for salad dressings, peanut or sesame for Asian stir fries.
- Spread your bread with margarine spreads made from vegetable oils, or avocado, low-fat dips and mayonnaise, peanut butter, ricotta or cottage cheese.

Eating goals for a healthier heart and blood vessels

Lower your intake of saturated fat, trans fat and cholesterol by:

- choosing lean meat and chicken
- replacing butter with margarine spreads using low-fat dairy products
- avoiding high-fat takeout, baked goods and processed snack foods
- eating less high-fat, processed deli meats

Balance your calorie intake with good portion control to maintain a healthy weight; eat more plant foods, especially legumes, nuts, seeds and brightly colored fruits and vegetables; choose high fiber, low glycemic index (GI) and whole grain carbohydrate foods; eat oily fish at least twice a week; use plant-sterol-enriched foods such as margarine, milk and yogurt; choose and prepare foods with less salt; and drink alcohol in moderation if at all.

Moderate dietary cholesterol

So, what about dietary cholesterol? The consensus is that while it's still important to keep cholesterol down, it's not as big a taboo as it once was.

The body of research now shows cholesterol from food can have little impact on your blood cholesterol levels, especially when your overall diet is good. Eggs, prawns and other crustaceans are also low in saturated fat and can be good sources of heart friendly omega-3 fats.

Moderation in dietary cholesterol does, however, remain the key. Expert opinion varies, but limiting your intake of eggs to three to four a week and having the occasional meal of shrimp cooked without added fat is unlikely to do most people with high cholesterol any harm. If you have familial hypercholesterolaemia or a very high risk of heart disease you are likely to be an exception to this advice and should take steps to be more strict with your cholesterol intake.

Health authorities recommend keeping total dietary cholesterol intake under 200–300 mg a day. Check our cholesterol ready chart on page 19 to see what that means for you.

Balance your calories

We live in a world where upsizing and "meal deals" are commonplace; quick-fix fad diets are bestsellers; and gadgets to save time and energy abound. It's no wonder we are in the midst of an obesity epidemic. Strategies to stop weight gain are essential in any heart-friendly eating plan and the most important of these are portion and calorie control. The equations to support this are simple: eat too much food and calories and you put on weight, eat less food and calories and you lose weight—or at the very least you won't gain. Despite the promises of diet books, there are no special foods or ways of eating that will change this basic equation. Physical activity is the only factor you can add to tip the balance in your favor.

Cutting back on your calories means focusing on foods that give you more for less—foods with more nutrients but less calories. Give foods like chips, commercial cakes, pastries and cookies, sweets, soft drinks and high-fat, savory crackers the flick and eat more fruit, vegetables, whole grain breads and cereals, lean meat, fish, nuts and seeds.

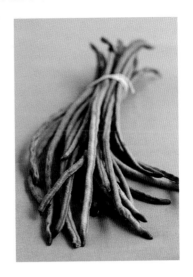

Watching the total amount of fat you eat also makes it easier to balance your calories. A no-fat diet is no good for lowering cholesterol (it's the balance of good fats and bad fats that counts) or losing weight for that matter (it just makes your diet unpalatable and hard to maintain), but eating less saturated fat will rid your diet of many unhealthy and surplus calories. Re-visit our tips for cutting back on saturated fat on page 15 to make sure you target the right ones.

Controlling portion sizes will also mean fewer calories. Try eating only the recommended serving of your cereal at breakfast—1⅓ cups of ready-to-eat cereal, ½ cup of natural muesli or 1 cup of cooked oatmeal—use a smaller sized plate or bowl for meals or order an entrée-sized meal if you must have a dessert when eating out. If you want seconds, go for another serving of salad or vegetables rather than the meat or the pasta/rice. Another trick to keeping portions in check is to divide up your plate at meal time—allow a quarter of the plate for your protein (such as meat), a quarter for your carbohydrate and the remaining half for salad or vegetables.

Choosing your carbohydrates wisely will also help with portion control. Select higher fiber, low-GI carbohydrates like grainy bread, pasta, oat-based breakfast cereals, sweet potato, corn, legumes and temperate fruits. Their slower digestion and absorption will keep you feeling fuller and satisfied for longer and make you less likely to snack before your next meal. Their soluble fiber also helps lower your blood cholesterol.

Statistics tell us that if you are overweight, you may never achieve your healthy weight goals despite your best attempts. If you do succeed, it can slip away again within three to five years with creeping weight gains. However, don't let this deter you.

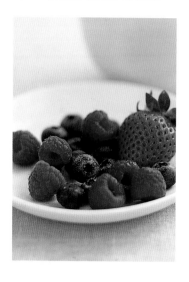

Any weight you lose will make you healthier and fitter. You only need a weight loss of around five to ten percent to make a positive difference to your cholesterol.

If you need more help with your weight and diet plan, visit a dietitian. They can help you with a heart-friendly eating plan to help you keep the pounds off.

Seek out antioxidants

Free radicals cause damage to your body—known as oxidation—which leads to aging and disease. When LDL cholesterol is oxidized by free radicals it becomes stickier and is more likely to take part in the process of atherosclerosis—this makes it more dangerous. You can prevent oxidation of LDL cholesterol by making sure you eat plenty of foods rich in antioxidants. Antioxidants are natural chemicals found in food that protect your body from damage by free radicals. Some antioxidants are also nutrients—think of vitamin C, E and selenium, while others are simply naturally occurring plant chemicals known as phytochemicals, such as the flavonoids, catechins and anthocyanins.

Color is a good sign of a food's health potential and most of the foods richest in antioxidant ability are also rich in color. Think of berries, citrus, cherries, plums, spinach and other green leafy vegetables, broccoli, red capsicum and beetroot.

Other antioxidant-rich foods include tea, red wine, chocolate, extra virgin olive oil, nuts and herbs.

Taking antioxidants out of food and putting them into a supplement can in some cases do you no good and may even do you harm. The safest and most effective way to get antioxidants is through food. What would you enjoy more, a bowl of fresh raspberries and a few squares of premium dark chocolate or a supplement pill?

Enjoy more plant foods

Research the world over reveals that people who eat the most fruit and vegetables are the healthiest and longest living of all. With most rich in cholesterol-lowering, soluble fiber and sterols, fruits and vegetables are also packed with heart-protective vitamins, minerals and antioxidants. With maximum nutrition, plant foods come at a very low kilojoule cost so are a great choice when you need to control your weight. To get the most from fruit and vegetables, eat by the rainbow. Choose at least two servings of fruit and five servings of vegetables each day, selecting the brightest and most colorful types to get maximum benefits.

Where's the cholesterol?	
Food	Cholesterol mg
Kidney, 100 g	500
Liver, 100 g	400
Egg, 1 large	210
Lobster, 100 g	150
Prawns, 100 g	110

Legumes are another important plant food. Be they fresh, dried or canned, legumes (for example, beans, split peas, chickpeas and lentils) are excellent sources of soluble fiber and low in saturated fat. Legumes are low in GI and rich in heart-friendly antioxidants that protect cholesterol from the oxidative damage that makes it more likely to clog up your arteries.

To reap the health rewards of legumes, incorporate them into at least a couple of meals a week. They make a great vegetarian alternative in curries (chickpeas) and Mexican dishes (kidney beans) but also serve up well at breakfast. You can also try cutting back the meat a little and adding them to stews and soups or using them to lower the GI of grains like rice and couscous.

Finally, don't forget nuts and seeds. Formerly considered to be off limits for anyone wanting a healthier diet, nuts and seeds have been given the thumbs up. While high in fats (the healthy kind) and calories, they are also rich in fiber, healthy fats and heart-protective nutrients like vitamin E, folate, magnesium and copper.

A small handful of unsalted nuts (raw, toasted or dry roasted) as a daily snack, or nuts and seeds added to salads, pasta or breakfast cereals are a good habit for a healthier heart. If you need to lose weight, include them only occasionally—up to a couple of times a week and always stop at just a small handful. Reassuringly, studies show those who eat nuts regularly are more likely to be a healthy weight.

Eat more fiber

Fiber is your friend when you need to get cholesterol down. Unfortunately most of us aren't friendly enough with fiber. Our intakes are often way down compared with the 25–30 g of fiber a day that's recommended.

Two types of fiber exist in food—soluble and insoluble. Both offer you plenty of health benefits, but it's the soluble fiber that directly affects blood cholesterol. Found in oats, barley, psyllium, legumes and some fruit and vegetables, soluble fiber forms a gel-like substance in your intestine that binds up cholesterol and stops your body absorbing it. Increase the soluble fiber in your diet by adding psyllium husk or oat, barley or rice bran to your breakfast cereal or baking recipes as well as making sure you eat enough fruit, vegetables and legumes.

Foods made from the whole of the grain—known as whole grain foods—are also rich in fiber (both soluble and insoluble), low in GI and packed with essential nutrients and antioxidants. The combination of goodies found in whole grains is responsible for their undisputed ability to protect not only from CVD but also diabetes, overweight and certain types of cancer.

Get the most out of these heart-friendly foods by making half of all the grain foods you eat whole grain. If you are aiming for six serves of cereal foods a day then at least three serves should be whole grain. The problem is, most of us are lucky to even make one serve, let alone three.

What fat is that?

Fat	Where will you find it?
Saturated fats	butter, cream, palm oil, coconut milk and cream, fried foods and take-aways, fat on meat and skin on chicken, full-fat dairy foods, deli meats and most commercial cakes, pastries, candy and cookies
Monounsaturated fats	olives and olive oil, avocados, peanuts and peanut oil, canola oil, macadamia nuts, hazelnuts, pecan nuts, cashews and almonds
Omega-6 polyunsaturated fats	sunflower, safflower, soy bean, sesame, cottonseed and grape seed oils, pine nuts and Brazil nuts
Omega-3 polyunsaturated fats	oily types of fish; herring, sardine, mackerel, salmon and tuna; walnuts, canola oil, flax seeds and linseed oil, lean red meat and a range of fortified commercial foods
Trans fats	margarines and fat spreads (some countries have less trans fats in these than others—check labels), deep-fried fast food, commercial cakes, pastries, pies and cookies—look for the words hydrogenated or partially hydrogenated fats on food labels

Whole grain foods aren't just "whole" grains like brown rice and whole-wheat. Whole grain foods can be processed and still retain the important components of the whole grain. Boost your daily serves of whole grain foods by:

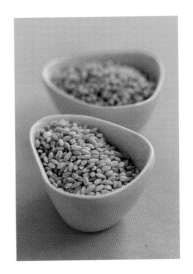

- using whole-wheat flour instead of white
- snacking on whole-wheat crackers or popcorn
- enjoying oats, natural muesli or whole-wheat cereals at breakfast
- choosing whole grain or wholemeal breads
- trying brown rice or barley as a change from white rice
- choosing wholemeal rather than white pasta

Eat more fish

Fish, especially oily fish contain healthy unsaturated fats known as long chain omega-3s. Omega-3 fats are a type of polyunsaturated fat that are essential to our health and must come from our diet. These fats protect the heart and blood vessels by lowering triglycerides, keeping the heart beating regularly (preventing arrhythmias), maintaining more elastic blood vessels, lessening the risk of blood clots by keeping the blood more free flowing, and calming inflammation.

To benefit most from omega-3, include oily fish at least twice a week. Highest concentrations of omega-3 can be found in sardines, salmon, mackerel, tuna, herring, trout, whitefish and bluefish. All fish, even the oily varieties, are low in saturated fat and so are a healthy choice at any meal.

It makes no difference if your fish is fresh or canned. The convenience of canned fish makes it perfect for busy lives and those who don't live near the sea. Take care to avoid fish packed in brine—you don't need the extra salt. Instead, look for canned fish packed in spring water and check the label for those with the most omega-3.

Consider plant sterols

Plant sterols are found naturally in plant-based foods such as vegetable oils, legumes, fruit, nuts and seeds. Able to reduce the amount of cholesterol your body absorbs from your intestine, plant sterols ultimately lower blood cholesterol. A typical Western

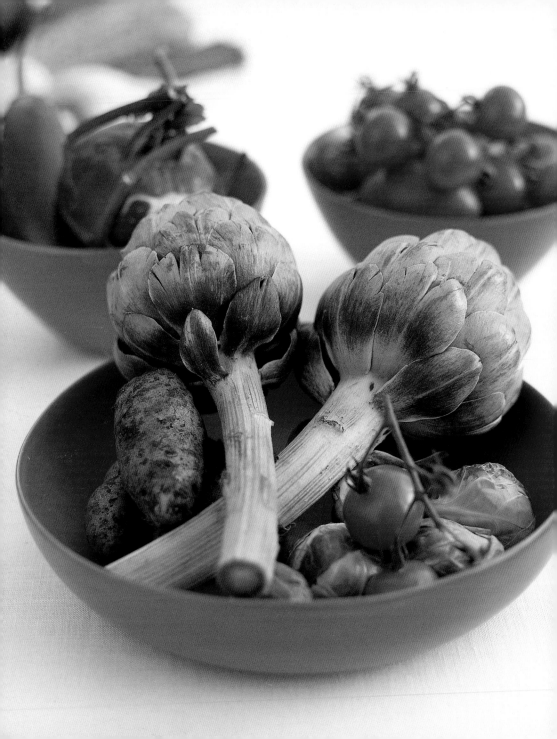

diet won't have enough plant sterols to make a difference to blood cholesterol but one that includes foods enriched with plant sterols will.

Depending upon where in the world you live, you may find margarine spreads, milk, yogurt and even breakfast cereals enriched with plant sterols. For blood cholesterol benefits you need to eat 2–3 g of plant sterols every day.

As a rule, three serves of a sterol-enriched food will give you enough plant sterols for the cholesterol-lowering benefits—check product packaging to be sure.

Sterol-enriched foods can't be expected to take the place of a healthy diet that is low in saturated fat. However, the weight of evidence is behind them and Heart Associations around the world recommend plant sterol-enriched foods be considered as part of a cholesterol lowering diet.

Up your oats
Oats are a food with a proven record for lowering cholesterol because of a soluble fiber known as beta glucan. But just don't eat any oats (though they are all good for you), go for the slower cooking, old fashioned varieties such as traditional, steel-cut or scotch oats, which will have a lower GI and more beta glucan than quick-cook and instant varieties.

Keep salt down

Although rising blood pressure as we age appears to be inevitable in the Western world, there are steps you can take to keep blood pressure in check. Losing weight, drinking less alcohol, being active and eating more fruit and vegetables will all help, as will cutting down on salt.

Around 75 percent of the salt we eat comes from processed foods. So simply avoiding salt in cooking or on the table is not enough. To get your salt intake down to healthier levels take care with what you bring home from the supermarket. Look for reduced-salt or no-added-salt varieties of the regular foods you buy, such as margarine spreads, canned tomatoes, tomato paste, tomato sauce, crackers, peanut butter, cheese, bread, and cooking stocks and sauces.

Avoiding obviously salty foods such as bacon, ham, olives, hard cheeses, canned fish in brine, salted nuts and chips will also help, as will using liberal amounts of fresh and dried herbs and spices to boost flavor and make the transition easier. Herbs and spices have added benefits besides the extra flavor—they are rich sources of health protective phytochemicals and antioxidants.

Drink alcohol in moderation

Research suggests that moderate alcohol consumption—a little regularly—can protect your heart and blood vessels. This is apparently the reason the French have such a good record for heart health. The United States Department of Health defines moderate or low-risk alcohol consumption as no more than two standard drinks a day. The American Heart Association also recommends no more than two drinks a day for men and one for women in its latest dietary and lifestyle recommendations to reduce CVD.

It also appears not to matter what you drink provided it is alcoholic. Beer, spirits, white wine or red, they all do a similar job—raising good HDL and keeping your blood flowing freely. Red wine with its antioxidants may offer a little extra benefit, but when all is said and done choose what you enjoy most and keep your intake modest.

Unfortunately, alcohol is a double-edged sword. Loaded with calories, alcohol is not good for your weight and too much raises your blood pressure and triglycerides—all of which increase your risk of heart disease. In excess, alcohol is also responsible for liver disease, some forms of cancer and early death by misadventure. For these reasons, if you don't already drink, don't start just to lower your risk of cardiovascular disease.

If you find it hard to just have one or two drinks try to:

- reduce your thirst with water or diet drinks before you drink alcohol
- choose low alcohol beer
- alternate alcoholic and non-alcoholic drinks
- dilute alcoholic drinks with soda or water.

Final words on lifestyle to lower cholesterol

Despite the fact that this is a cookbook, advice about lowering cholesterol and improving heart health is not complete without mentioning the importance of a healthy lifestyle. Giving up smoking and becoming more physically active are essential for keeping your heart—and the rest of your body—healthy.

Sitting around like a couch potato makes you twice as likely to die of a heart attack as someone who regularly exercises. Continuing to smoke means a heart attack is up to six times more likely for you than for someone who doesn't smoke.

Taking up the lifestyle challenge offers impressive results: within just one year of quitting smoking, heart disease risk drops by 50 percent, and if you are overweight but fit, your risk of early death drops to around one-third that of your equally heavy but unfit peers. What's more, those that have the most to gain from moving more are those who are currently doing the least.

Contact your local "quit smoking" services to start the ball rolling toward going smoke free. These services can give you the best advice about when and how to start to quit plus support and motivation to keep you going once you are on your way.

Before tackling your fitness regimen discuss your plans with your doctor. This is especially important if you haven't exercised regularly for a while or have other health problems. When you have the all-clear, aim to build up to 30 minutes of moderate intensity activity on most, if not all, days of the week. Moderate intensity means you are breathing a little harder, but you can still chat with a friend.

If you are new to the whole exercise thing, consider a few sessions with a personal trainer or exercise physiologist. They can design a program that suits your health needs best.

Your 30 minutes doesn't have to be continuous either. Research shows three 10-minute sessions offer the same benefits as one 30-minute session. Thirty minutes is also the bare minimum you need for health. If you are up to it, and can do more, then there are only greater health benefits to gain. To lose weight you need to do at least 60 minutes of exercise a day.

Consider these ways to be more physically active in your life:

- invest in a pedometer and work towards more steps (or 7500–10,000 steps a day if you are up to the challenge)
- take the stairs rather than the elevator or escalator
- park a little further away from the entrance to your work or the shopping mall
- walk to get the paper rather than taking the car
- get up to turn the TV off rather than using the remote
- make a regular date with a friend to go for a walk
- hop on your bike and go for a ride or invest in an exercise bike—you can get at least 30–60 minutes just watching your favorite TV show
- join a water aerobics group—this is good if you have joint problems or are very overweight
- take up a physical hobby like line dancing, yoga, swimming, tennis or golf
- enjoy active weekends with family and friends: go to the park for a picnic and a game of Frisbee, go bushwalking or take a visit to the city for some sightseeing.

How to use this book

The tested recipes in this book have been selected to offer you a range of heart-healthy meals and snacks that can be enjoyed by everyone. Switching the whole family to healthier eating means everyone benefits—especially children. Good habits are learned young—just don't forget children under 2 years should continue with their full-fat dairy foods. From 2 years, introduce the lower fat products the rest of the family use.

There are recipes for everyday meals as well as special occasions and all aim for less saturated fat. To push the benefits of these recipes further we have included low-salt, high-fiber, low-GI and whole grain ingredients wherever possible. We have also tried to include more heart-protective foods such as oats, legumes, nuts, brightly colored fruits and vegetables, and fish, so you get the most for your heart and blood vessels from each recipe.

Note: Many recipes call for self-rising flour. If you cannot find this in your supermarket, you can use all-purpose flour and add 1 ½ teaspoons baking powder for each cup of flour used.

Disclaimer
The information in this book is intended to provide people with high cholesterol, and people who care for them, with general advice about healthy low-cholesterol eating (accurate at the time of printing). This advice may not be sufficient for some people with multiple health problems or serious complications. It is not intended to replace any advice given to you by a qualified doctor or other mainstream health professional. It is important that high cholesterol is diagnosed by a doctor, using standard diagnostic tests (such as blood tests). Neither the author nor the publishers can be held responsible for claims arising from the inappropriate use or incorrect interpretation of any of the dietary advice described in this book.

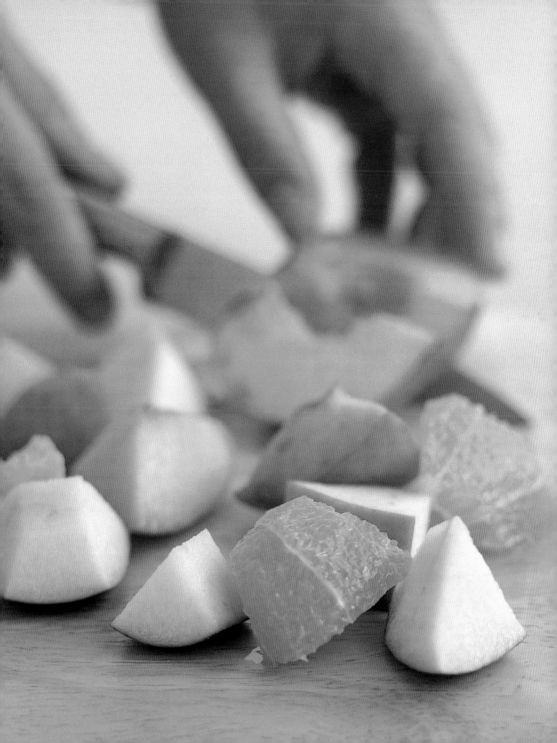

BREAKFAST

MUESLI BOOST

GET YOURSELF OFF TO AN ENERGY-FUELLED START TO THE DAY WITH THIS NUTRITIOUS MUESLI—RICH IN CARBOHYDRATE, FIBER, B-GROUP VITAMINS, BETA-CAROTENE, POTASSIUM AND MAGNESIUM.

1/3 **cup flaked almonds**
2 cups rolled oats
1 cup processed bran cereal
1/3 **cup rye flakes**
1/4 **cup pepitas**
2 tbsp sunflower seeds
1 tbsp flax seeds
3/4 **cup golden raisins**

1 cup chopped dried apricots
1/2 **cup chopped dried pear**
low-fat honey-flavored yogurt or skim milk, to serve

PREP TIME: 10 MINUTES
COOKING TIME: 5 MINUTES
SERVINGS: 6

Preheat the oven to 315°F. Put the almonds on a baking tray in a single layer and toast in the oven for 5 minutes, or until golden. Remove and set aside.

Put the rolled oats, processed bran cereal, rye flakes, pumpkin, sunflower and flax seeds in a bowl, then stir well to combine. Add the raisins, apricots and pears as well as the toasted almonds.

Serve with low-fat honey-flavored yogurt or skim milk.

HINT:
• Any remaining muesli can be kept in an airtight container for up to 2 weeks.

nutrition per serving: Energy 433 Cal; Fat 11.8 g; Saturated fat 1.5 g; Protein 11.2 g; Carbohydrate 65.9 g; Fiber 13.1 g; Cholesterol 0 mg; Sodium 61 mg

BIRCHER MUESLI

THIS DELICIOUS MUESLI, WITH THE ADDED BENEFIT OF FRESH FRUIT, IS
A GREAT ALTERNATIVE TO REGULAR MUESLI. IT'S RICH IN CARBOHYDRATES
AND CONTAINS MOST VITAMINS AND MINERALS.

3 cups rolled oats
1 cup low-fat milk
⅓ cup low-fat plain yogurt
½ cup orange juice
3 tbsp sugar
½ cup low-fat plain
yogurt, extra
2 apples, grated

2 cups mixed seasonal fresh fruit (banana,
peach, apricot, melon, apple, strawberries)
honey, to serve (optional)

PREP TIME: 15 MINUTES + 4 HOURS
  REFRIGERATION
COOKING TIME: NONE
SERVINGS: 6

Put the oats, milk, yogurt, orange juice and sugar in a bowl and mix together well.
Cover and refrigerate for 4 hours, or overnight. Serve with the extra yogurt, grated
apple and fresh fruit of your choice. Drizzle with a little honey, if desired.

HINT:
• You can also add ½ cup slivered almonds, if you like. This will increase
  the fat and energy content, but the fat will be mostly the unsaturated type.

nutrition per serving: Energy 305 Cal; Fat 4.5 g; Saturated fat 0.8 g; Protein 10.3 g; Carbohydrate
52.8 g; Fiber 5.5 g; Cholesterol 4 mg; Sodium 55 mg

MIXED BERRY COUSCOUS

1 cup instant couscous

2 cups unsweetened apple and cranberry juice

1 cinnamon stick

2 cups raspberries

1²/₃ cups blueberries

1²/₃ cups strawberries, hulled and halved

2 tsp lime or lemon zest, plus extra, to serving

1 tbsp finely shredded mint

7 oz low-fat plain or fruit-flavored yogurt

2 tbsp pure maple syrup

PREP TIME: 10 MINUTES + STANDING + REFRIGERATION TIME

COOKING TIME: 5 MINUTES

SERVINGS: 4

Put the couscous in a bowl. Pour the juice into a small saucepan and add the cinnamon stick. Bring to a boil, then remove from the heat and pour over the couscous. Cover with plastic wrap and leave to stand for 5 minutes, or until the liquid has been absorbed. Remove the cinnamon stick. Refrigerate.

Separate the couscous grains with a fork, add the berries, lime zest and mint, and gently fold through. Spoon the mixture into 4 bowls. Top with a large dollop of plain or fruit-flavored yogurt and drizzle with the maple syrup. Serve chilled.

HINT:
• You can make this dish with many other great fruit combinations, including orange juice and dried fruits or fresh mango, peach, pear and apple.

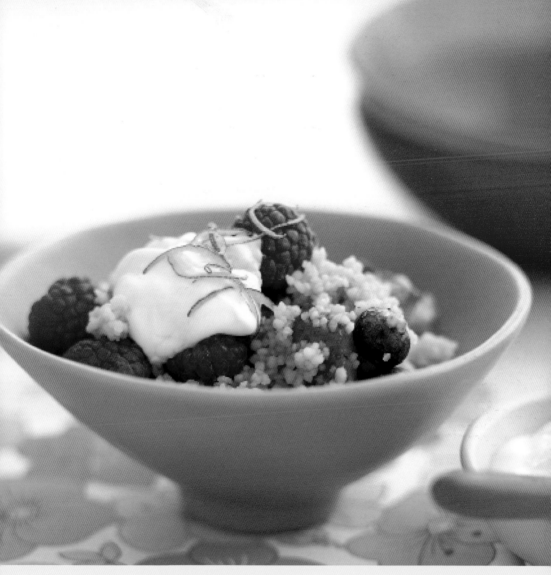

THIS TASTY, LOW-GI BREAKFAST IS
PACKED WITH FRESH SUMMER
FRUIT AND ZESTY SPICES. IT IS A
GOOD SOURCE OF VITAMIN C AND
RICH IN ANTIOXIDANTS.

nutrition per serving: Energy 364 Cal
Fat 0.8 g
Saturated fat 0.1 g
Protein 11.2 g
Carbohydrate 73.2 g
Fiber 6.6 g
Cholesterol 2 mg
Sodium 58 mg

OATMEAL WITH STEWED RHUBARB

INCLUDING RHUBARB IN THIS OATMEAL MAKES THIS BREAKFAST EVEN
MORE NUTRITIOUS THAN REGULAR OATMEAL—ADDING VITAMIN C, CALCIUM,
POTASSIUM AND DIETARY FIBER.

DRY OATMEAL MIX
6 cups rolled oats
½ cup rolled rice flakes
½ cup rolled barley
½ cup rolled rye
¼ cup millet flakes

STEWED RHUBARB
¾ rhubarb, trimmed and washed
½ cup brown sugar
¼ tsp pumpkin pie spice
low-fat yogurt, to serve

PREP TIME: 15 MINUTES
COOKING TIME: 30 MINUTES
SERVINGS: 4

Put all the oatmeal ingredients in a large bowl and mix together well. The dry mix makes about 8 cups or enough for 16 servings. Store in a large airtight container for up to 2 months.

To make enough porridge for 4 servings, put 2 cups porridge mixture in a saucepan with 5 cups water. Bring to a boil, then reduce the heat and simmer, stirring frequently, over a medium heat for 15 minutes, or until the porridge is thick.
If it is too thick, add a little skim milk or water.

Meanwhile, to make the stewed rhubarb, chop the rhubarb into ¾ in lengths.
Put in a saucepan with the sugar, spice and 1 cup water. Slowly bring to a boil, stirring to dissolve the sugar, then reduce the heat and simmer for
10 minutes, stirring often. Serve hot or cold with the porridge.

HINTS:
- The cooking time of the porridge will decrease considerably if you use quick-cooking oats (one-minute oats). Check the labels on the packets before purchase. However, quick-cooking oats have a higher GI value than slower-cooking ones.
- If you have trouble finding some of these ingredients in your local supermarket, look for them at a good health food shop.

nutrition per serving: Energy 297 Cal; Fat 3.7 g; Saturated fat 0.6 g; Protein 6 g; Carbohydrate 59 g; Fiber 4.7 g; Cholesterol 0 mg; Sodium 10 mg

POACHED DRIED FRUIT WITH WHOLE SPICES

THIS FRUIT COMPOTE IS A LITTLE DIFFERENT FROM OTHER FRUIT COMPOTES WITH THE EXOTIC TOUCH OF ADDED SPICES.

1 orange
1 lemon
1 cup unsweetened apple juice
6 whole cardamom pods, lightly crushed
6 whole cloves
1 cinnamon stick
13 oz dried-fruit medley
3 tbsp brown sugar

PREP TIME: 10 MINUTES + 1 HOUR SOAKING
TOTAL COOKING TIME: 15 MINUTES
SERVINGS: 8

Peel 3 large strips of orange rind, avoiding too much white pith. Peel the lemon rind into thick strips. Cut half the orange and lemon rinds into thin strips.

Put the apple juice, whole spices and thick strips of rind in a large saucepan with 3 cups water and bring to a boil. Add the dried fruit. Remove from the heat and set aside for 1 hour.

Return to the heat, add the brown sugar and thin strips of rind and cover. Cook over low heat for 5 minutes, or until soft. Remove the fruit with a slotted spoon. Simmer the juice for another 5 minutes, or until reduced and thickened slightly. Serve the fruit warm or cold drizzled with juice.

HINT:
• This will keep well for at least a week covered and refrigerated.

nutrition per serving: Energy 150 Cal; Fat 0.2 g; Saturated fat 0 g; Protein 1.4 g; Carbohydrate 35 g; Fiber 3.7 g; Cholesterol 0 mg; Sodium 13 mg

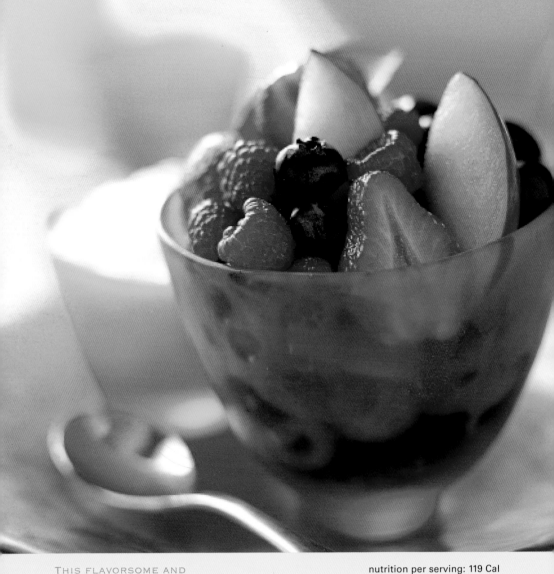

THIS FLAVORSOME AND
COLORFUL FRUIT SALAD
CONTAINS AN ASSORTMENT
OF BERRIES, AND IS LADEN
WITH THE GOODNESS OF
VITAMINS, ANTIOXIDANTS
AND PHYTOCHEMICALS.

nutrition per serving: 119 Cal
Fat 0.3 g
Saturated fat 0 g
Protein 1.9 g
Carbohydrate 24.9 g
Fiber 4.4 g
Cholesterol 0 mg
Sodium 6 mg

RED FRUIT SALAD WITH BERRIES

SYRUP
¼ cup sugar
½ cup unsweetened apple and
 cranberry juice
1 star anise
1 tsp finely chopped lemon rind

1²/₃ cups strawberries, hulled and halved
1 cup blueberries
1¼ cups raspberries, mulberries or other
 red berries
1¼ cups pitted cherries

5 small red plums, about 9 oz, pits
 removed and quartered
low-fat yogurt, to serve (optional)

PREP TIME: 5 MINUTES +
 30 MINUTES COOLING +
 30 MINUTES REFRIGERATION
TOTAL COOKING TIME: 5 MINUTES
SERVINGS: 6

To make the syrup, put the sugar, juice, star anise, lemon rind and ½ cup water in a small saucepan. Bring to a boil over medium heat, stirring to dissolve the sugar. Boil the syrup for 3 minutes, then set aside to cool for 30 minutes. When cool, strain the syrup.

Mix the fruit together in a large bowl and pour on the syrup. Mix well to coat the fruit in the syrup and refrigerate until cooled. Serve the fruit dressed with a little syrup and the yogurt.

MUSHROOMS WITH SCRAMBLED EGGS AND WHOLEGRAIN BREAD

THIS IS A WHOLESOME, NOURISHING BREAKFAST, AND A GREAT WAY TO START THE DAY. IT PROVIDES GOOD AMOUNTS OF TOP-QUALITY PROTEIN, VITAMIN A, IRON AND FOLATE.

4 field mushrooms
olive oil spray
4 roma (plum) tomatoes, halved
3 tbsp balsamic vinegar
4 eggs, lightly beaten
4 egg whites, lightly beaten
3 tbsp low-fat milk

2 tbsp snipped fresh chives
8 thick slices wholegrain bread

PREP TIME: 15 MINUTES
COOKING TIME: 15 MINUTES
SERVINGS: 4

Trim the mushroom stalks to ¾ in below the cap. Wipe the mushrooms with paper towels to remove any dirt and grit.

Spray both sides of the mushrooms with the oil and place on a non-stick baking tray with the tomatoes. Drizzle the mushrooms and tomatoes with the balsamic vinegar, then season with freshly ground black pepper and place under a medium grill (broiler) for 10–15 minutes, or until tender.

Meanwhile, put the eggs, egg whites, milk and chives in a bowl and whisk together to combine. Pour the mixture into a non-stick frying pan and cook over low heat for 2–3 minutes, or until the egg begins to set, then gently stir with a wooden spoon to scramble.

Toast the wholegrain bread until golden brown, then cut diagonally. Serve with the mushrooms, tomato and scrambled eggs.

HINT:
• Use omega-3-enriched eggs instead of regular eggs to get more of the essential omega-3 fatty acids. Omega-3-enriched eggs are available in most large supermarkets and some health food shops.

nutrition per serving: Energy 334 Cal; Fat 8.5 g; Saturated fat 2 g; Protein 20.8 g; Carbohydrate 39.5 g; Fiber 6.1 g; Cholesterol 188 mg; Sodium 572 mg

CORN CAKES WITH TOMATO SALSA

THESE TASTY CORN CAKES ARE A GREAT TREAT TO HAVE ON THE WEEKEND.
THE TOMATO SALSA CONTAINS VITAMINS C AND E, AND BETA-CAROTENE.

TOMATO SALSA
2 tbsp diced red onion
2 firm tomatoes, seeded and diced
1/2 cucumber, seeded
  and diced
2 tbsp flat-leaf (Italian) parsley, chopped
1 tbsp olive oil
1 tbsp white vinegar

4 fresh corn cobs or 15 oz can corn kernels,
  drained
2 spring onions (scallions), finely chopped
2 eggs, lightly beaten
1 1/4 cups self-rising flour
3/4 cup low-fat milk
olive oil spray

PREP TIME: 15 MINUTES
TOTAL COOKING TIME: 15 MINUTES
SERVINGS: 4

To make the tomato salsa, put the red onion, tomato, cucumber and parsley in a bowl. Season with freshly ground black pepper, then add the oil and vinegar and toss together well to coat.

If using fresh corn, remove the kernels by cutting down the length of the cob with a sharp knife. Put the kernels in a small bowl with the spring onion and combine.

Whisk together the egg, self-rising flour and milk in a bowl until smooth. Fold in the corn and spring onion mixture and season to taste with freshly ground black pepper.

Heat a frying pan over medium heat and spray with oil. Working in batches, drop 1/4 cup of batter per corn cake into the pan and allow enough space for spreading. Cook over medium heat for 2 minutes, or until golden. Turn over and cook for a further 1–2 minutes, or until golden. Repeat with the remaining batter to make 12 corn cakes.

To serve, stack three corn cakes on individual plates and top with some tomato salsa.

nutrition per serving: Energy 345 Cal; Fat 9.4 g; Saturated fat 1.7 g; Protein 12.8 g; Carbohydrate 48.8 g; Fiber 5.4 g; Cholesterol 96 mg; Sodium 347 mg

BANANA BREAD WITH MAPLE RICOTTA

1/3 cup strong coffee

2/3 cup brown sugar

1 egg

1 egg white

3 tbsp canola oil

1 tsp vanilla extract

3 ripe bananas, mashed

1 cup all-purpose flour

2 cups self-rising flour

1/2 tsp baking powder

1 tsp ground ginger

1/2 tsp ground nutmeg

1 tsp ground cinnamon

1 tsp baking soda

7 oz low-fat ricotta cheese

2 tbsp maple syrup

fresh berries, to serve

PREP TIME: 10 MINUTES

COOKING TIME: 55 MINUTES

MAKES 10–12 SLICES

Preheat the oven to 325°F. Lightly grease a 8½ x 4½ in loaf pan and line the base with baking paper. Heat the coffee in a small saucepan over low heat, add the brown sugar and stir until the sugar has dissolved.

Put the egg, egg white, oil and vanilla in a bowl and beat until just combined. Add the coffee mixture and banana.

Sift the flours, baking powder, ginger, nutmeg, cinnamon and baking soda onto the mixture and stir gently to combine—do not overbeat. Spoon the mixture into the prepared loaf pan. Bake for 50 minutes, or until a skewer comes out clean when inserted into the center. Leave in the tin for 10 minutes before turning out onto a wire rack to cool completely.

Combine the ricotta and maple syrup in a small bowl. Cut the banana bread into thick slices and serve with the maple ricotta and fresh berries.

HINT:
• Any leftover banana bread can be frozen in an airtight container with pieces of baking paper between each slice.

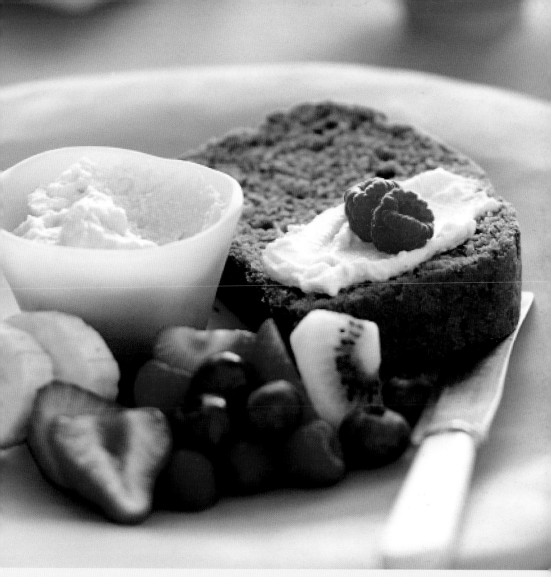

THIS REDUCED-FAT BANANA BREAD
IS A GREAT DISH TO SERVING FOR
BRUNCH. IT PROVIDES
CARBOHYDRATES, PROTEIN AND
MINERALS, AND THE MAPLE
RICOTTA AND BERRIES GIVE THE
ADDED BENEFIT OF CALCIUM,
FIBER AND ANTIOXIDANTS.

nutrition per slice (12): Energy 267 Cal
Fat 6.4 g
Saturated fat 0.9 g
Protein 7.3 g
Carbohydrate 43.6 g
Fiber 3.6 g
Cholesterol 16 mg
Sodium 348 mg

OATY BUCKWHEAT PANCAKES

THESE DELICIOUS PANCAKES ARE ALSO NUTRITIOUS. THEY CONTAIN SLOWLY DIGESTED CARBOHYDRATES, FIBER AND PROTEIN, AND THE BERRIES ARE RICH IN VITAMINS AND ANTIOXIDANTS.

BERRY SAUCE
¼ cup sugar
2 tsp lemon juice
2 cups raspberries

⅓ cup buckwheat flour
⅔ cup whole-wheat flour
1½ tsp baking powder
¼ cup rolled oats
1 egg yolk

1½ cups buttermilk
3 egg whites
olive or canola oil spray
extra raspberries, to serve

PREP TIME: 15 MINUTES
COOKING TIME: 40 MINUTES
SERVINGS: 4

To make the sauce, put the sugar, lemon juice and ¼ cup water in a saucepan over medium heat and bring to a boil. Add the raspberries and cook over low heat for 3 minutes. Cool, then purée in a food processor or blender for 10 seconds.

Sift the flours into a bowl and return the husks to the bowl. Add the baking powder and rolled oats and combine. Make a well in the center. Combine the egg yolk and buttermilk and add to the dry ingredients all at once. Stir to form a smooth batter. Whisk the egg whites until firm peaks form, then fold into the batter.

Heat a frying pan over medium heat and spray with oil. Pour ¼ cup batter into the pan and swirl to form a 4 in circle. Cook for 1–2 minutes, or until bubbles appear on the surface. Turn and cook for 1–2 minutes, or until light brown. Transfer to a plate and keep warm. Repeat to make 8 pancakes. Serve with the berry sauce and raspberries.

nutrition per serving: Energy 323 Cal; Fat 5.9 g; Saturated fat 2 g; Protein 13.3 g; Carbohydrate 49.5 g; Fiber 8 g; Cholesterol 53 mg; Sodium 368 mg

FRUIT FRAPPE

THIS DRINK IS A REFRESHING ANTIOXIDANT BREAKFAST COCKTAIL, RICH IN VITAMIN C, BETA-CAROTENE AND FIBER. IT'S ALSO LOW IN SODIUM AND HIGH IN POTASSIUM, WHICH IS GOOD FOR BLOOD PRESSURE CONTROL.

10 dried apricot halves
1½ cups raspberries
1 banana, roughly chopped
1 mango, chopped
2 cups orange juice
1 tbsp mint leaves
6 ice cubes

PREP TIME: 5 MINUTES + 10 MINUTES SOAKING
COOKING TIME: NONE
SERVINGS: 4

Put the dried apricots in a heatproof bowl. Cover with ¼ cup boiling water and soak for 10 minutes, or until plump. Drain, then roughly chop.

Put the chopped apricots, raspberries, banana, mango, orange juice, mint leaves and ice cubes in a blender, and blend until thick and smooth.

nutrition per serving: Energy 139 Cal; Fat 0.5 g; Saturated fat 0 g; Protein 2.6 g; Carbohydrate 28.1 g; Fiber 5.2 g; Cholesterol 0 mg; Sodium 13 mg

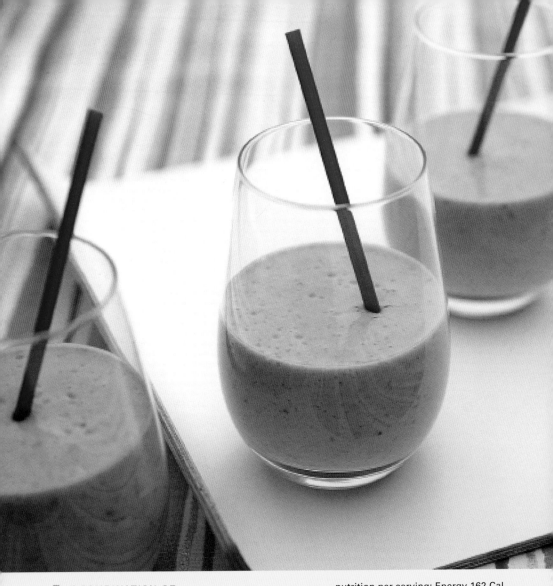

THE COMBINATION OF
RASPBERRIES AND BANANAS
MAKES THIS DRINK RICH IN
SOLUBLE FIBER, WHICH CAN
HELP LOWER CHOLESTEROL
WHEN CONSUMED REGULARLY.

nutrition per serving: Energy 162 Cal
Fat 0.6 g
Saturated fat 0.2 g
Protein 10.3 g
Carbohydrate 27 g
Fiber 3.2 g
Cholesterol 8 mg
Sodium 109 mg

LOW-FAT RASPBERRY AND BANANA SMOOTHIE

2½ cups skim milk

2 bananas

1 cup raspberries

¾ cup low-fat vanilla yogurt

1 tbsp oat bran

PREP TIME: 5 MINUTES + 30 MINUTES
 CHILLING

COOKING TIME: NONE

SERVINGS: 4

Put the milk in a covered container in the freezer for 30 minutes to make it very cold. It should be cold but not icy.

Peel and chop the bananas and put them in a blender. Add the raspberries, yogurt, oat bran and 1 cup of the milk. Blend for 30 seconds, or until smooth.

Add the remaining milk and blend for a further 30 seconds, or until combined. Pour into four glasses and serve immediately.

CARROT COCKTAIL

THIS DRINK IS AN EASY WAY TO BOOST YOUR NUTRIENT INTAKE AND TASTES MUCH BETTER THAN A VITAMIN SUPPLEMENT. IT IS RICH IN BETA-CAROTENE AND POTASSIUM, AND ALSO PROVIDES SOME FOLATE AND NIACIN.

10–12 carrots, quartered lengthways
½ cup pineapple juice
½ cup unsweetened orange juice
1–2 tsp honey, to taste
8 ice cubes

PREP TIME: 10 MINUTES
COOKING TIME: NONE
SERVINGS: 2

Using the plunger, push the carrot pieces through a juicer.

Combine the carrot juice with the pineapple juice, orange juice, honey and ice cubes in a jug and serve.

nutrition per serving: Energy 171 Cal; Fat 0.5 g; Saturated fat 0 g; Protein 3.2 g; Carbohydrate 33.7 g; Fiber 8 g; Cholesterol 0 mg; Sodium 156 mg

PEACH AND CANTALOUPE JUICE

A REFRESHING THIRST QUENCHER, THIS DRINK PROVIDES SWEET NATURAL SUGAR FOR ENERGY AND A BOOST OF VITAMIN C, BETA-CAROTENE, FOLATE, POTASSIUM AND FIBER.

½ cantaloupe
4 peaches
21 fl oz unsweetened orange juice
12 ice cubes
1 tbsp lime juice

PREP TIME: 10 MINUTES
COOKING TIME: NONE
SERVINGS: 2

Peel the cantaloupe, remove the seeds and roughly chop the flesh into bite-sized pieces. Cut a cross in the base of each peach. Put them in a heatproof bowl and cover with boiling water. Leave for 1–2 minutes, then remove with a slotted spoon, cool slightly and peel. Halve, remove the pit, and chop the flesh into bite-sized pieces.

Put the fruit in a blender with the orange juice and ice cubes, and blend until smooth. If the juice is too thick, add a little iced water. Stir in the lime juice and serve immediately.

nutrition per serving: Energy 235 Cal; Fat 0.8 g; Saturated fat 0 g; Protein 4.6 g; Carbohydrate 47.9 g; Fiber 5 g; Cholesterol 0 mg; Sodium 38 mg

SUMMER FRUIT SOY SMOOTHIE

1 banana

4 peaches, chopped

¾ cup apricot and mango soy yogurt or
   vanilla soy yogurt

1 tbsp oat bran

1 tsp natural vanilla extract

2½ cups reduced-fat plain soy milk or
   vanilla soy milk

1 tbsp maple syrup, optional

extra peach slices, to serve

ice cubes, to serve

PREP TIME: 10 MINUTES

COOKING TIME: NONE

SERVINGS: 4

Put the banana, peach, yogurt, oat bran, vanilla extract and 1 cup of the soy milk in a blender and blend for 30 seconds, or until smooth.

Add the remaining soy milk and blend for a further 30 seconds, or until combined. Taste for sweetness and add the maple syrup, if using. Put the ice and extra peach slices in four glasses, pour in the smoothie and serve immediately.

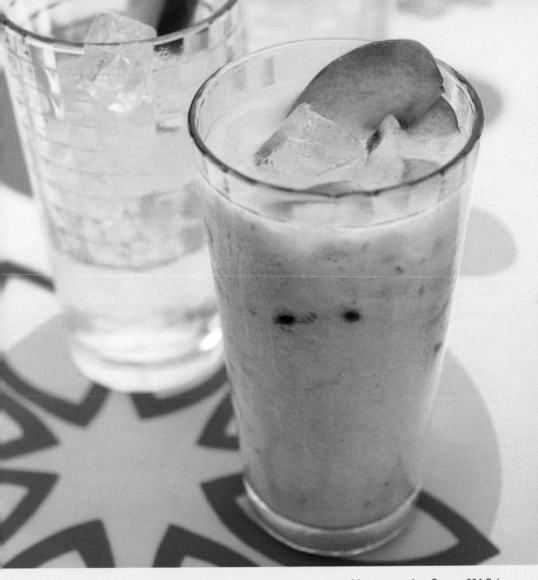

THIS SOY SMOOTHIE IS LOW
IN CHOLESTEROL AND A GOOD
CHOICE FOR PEOPLE WHO
CAN'T TOLERATE DAIRY
PRODUCTS. USE CALCIUM-
ENRICHED SOY MILK FOR AN
EXTRA CALCIUM BOOST.

nutrition per serving: Energy 224 Cal
Fat 1.9 g
Saturated fat 0.3 g
Protein 9.4 g
Carbohydrate 37.9 g
Fiber 4.5 g
Cholesterol 0 mg
Sodium 78 mg

SNACKS AND STARTERS

WHITE BEAN, CHICKPEA AND HERB DIP

THIS DELICIOUS DIP CONTAINS LESS FAT AND CALORIES THAN COMMERCIAL CREAM-BASED DIPS AND IS GREAT TO SNACK ON OR SERVE AT PARTIES AND BARBECUES. IT IS AN EASY WAY TO EAT MORE LEGUMES AND VEGETABLES.

3 slices wholegrain bread

3 tbsp low-fat milk

14 oz can cannellini beans, drained and rinsed

10½ oz can chickpeas, drained and rinsed

2 spring onions (scallions), finely chopped

⅓ cup low-fat plain yogurt

2 tbsp lemon juice

2 tsp finely-grated lemon zest

1 tbsp chopped parsley

2 tsp chopped oregano

1 tbsp olive oil

vegetable crudités, to serve

PREP TIME: 10 MINUTES

COOKING TIME: NONE

SERVINGS: 12

Remove the crusts from the bread, put the bread in a bowl and drizzle with the milk. Leave for 2 minutes, then mash with your fingertips until very soft.

Using a food processor or blender, process the cannellini beans, chickpeas, soaked bread, spring onion, yogurt, lemon juice, zest, herbs and oil until combined but retaining some texture. Season well with freshly ground black pepper. Serve at room temperature with the vegetable crudités.

HINT:
• To make vegetable crudités, cut raw carrots, celery, zucchini and unpeeled cucumbers into 2¾ in sticks and raw cauliflower and broccoli into small florets.

nutrition per serving: Energy 75 Cal; Fat 2.2 g; Saturated fat 0.3 g; Protein 4 g; Carbohydrate 8.7 g; Fiber 2.7 g; Cholesterol 1 mg; Sodium 60 mg

PATE WITH TORTILLA CRISPS

WITH FAR LESS FAT THAN POTATO CHIPS AND REGULAR PÂTÉ, THIS SNACK IS
A GOOD OPTION WHEN YOU'RE LOOKING FOR SOMETHING SAVORY AND
CRUNCHY TO NIBBLE ON.

1 tsp olive oil

1 small onion, chopped

2 garlic cloves, crushed

10½ oz flat mushrooms, wiped clean and
chopped

4 tbsp white wine or water

1 cup fresh whole-wheat breadcrumbs

2 tbsp finely chopped thyme, plus extra to
serve

2 tbsp chopped flat-leaf (Italian) parsley

1 tbsp lemon juice

4 large tortillas, about 8 in in diameter,
each cut into 8 wedges

olive oil spray

PREP TIME: 15 MINUTES + 1 HOUR
REFRIGERATION

COOKING TIME: 20 MINUTES

SERVINGS: 4–6

Heat the oil in a large, deep frying pan. Add the onion and garlic and cook, stirring, for
2 minutes without browning. Add the mushrooms and wine. Cook, stirring for 1 minute,
then cover and simmer for 5 minutes, stirring once or twice. Remove the lid and increase
the heat to evaporate any liquid. Cool.

Put the mushroom mixture, breadcrumbs, herbs and lemon juice in a food processor or
blender. Process until smooth and season well with freshly ground black pepper. Spoon
into a serving bowl. Cover and refrigerate for at least 1 hour to allow the flavors to develop.

Preheat the oven to 350°F. Put the tortilla wedges on a large baking tray and lightly spray
with the oil. Lightly sprinkle with freshly ground black pepper. Bake for 8 minutes, or until
crisp. Serve the pâté with the tortilla chips.

HINTS:
- Three slices of wholemeal (whole-wheat) bread, crusts removed, will yield about 1 cup
  of crumbs.
- Left-over tortilla chips can be stored in the freezer for up to 1 month. Re-crisp them in a
  325°F oven for 5 minutes.

nutrition per serving (6): Energy 144 Cal; Fat 3.4 g; Saturated fat 0.5 g; Protein 5.5 g; Carbohydrate
18.8 g; Fiber 3.7 g; Cholesterol 0 mg; Sodium 181 mg

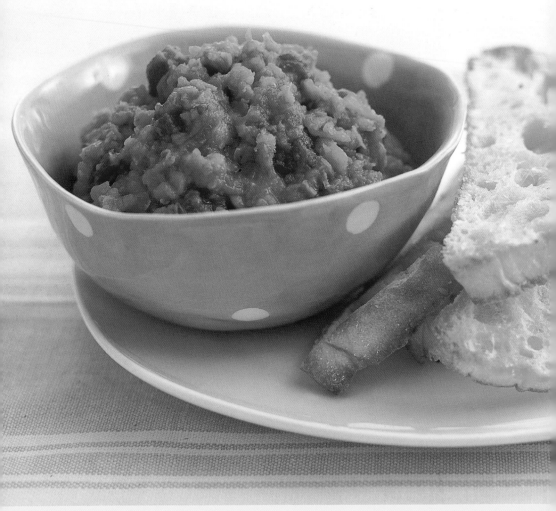

THIS TASTY DIP IS A GOOD WAY
TO INCLUDE LEGUMES IN YOUR
DIET. IT'S RELATIVELY LOW
IN CALORIES AND IS A RICH
SOURCE OF THE ANTIOXIDANT
BETA-CAROTENE.

nutrition per serving (8): Energy 92 Cal
Fat 1.9 g
Saturated fat 0.3 g
Protein 5.4 g
Carbohydrate 11.9 g
Fiber 3.2 g
Cholesterol 1 mg
Sodium 164 mg

SWEET POTATO AND RED LENTIL DIP

2 tsp olive oil
1 small red onion, finely chopped
1 garlic clove, crushed
1 tsp grated fresh ginger
1 tbsp Thai red curry paste
7 oz canned reduced-salt
   diced tomatoes
½ cup red lentils, drained
   and rinsed

1½ cups reduced-salt chicken stock
1 medium sweet potato,
   roughly chopped

PREP TIME: 20 MINUTES + COOLING TIME
COOKING TIME: 50 MINUTES
SERVINGS: 6–8

Heat the oil in a saucepan over medium heat and cook the onion for 2 minutes, or until softened. Add the garlic, ginger and curry paste and stir for 30 seconds.

Add the tomatoes, lentils and stock to the pan. Bring to a boil, then reduce the heat to low, cover and simmer, stirring often, for 30 minutes, or until the mixture thickens and the lentils have softened but are still intact. Spoon the mixture into a bowl and refrigerate until cold.

Meanwhile, put the sweet potato in a steamer and cover with a lid. Sit the steamer over a wok or saucepan of boiling water and steam for 15 minutes, or until tender. Transfer to a bowl, cool and mash roughly with a fork.

Carefully stir the mashed sweet potato into the lentil mixture with a fork. Season to taste with freshly ground black pepper. Serve with pita bread wedges, savory crackers or crusty bread for dipping.

BEETROOT HUMMUS

THIS LOW-GI DIP CONTAINS GOOD AMOUNTS OF FIBER, FOLATE, POTASSIUM AND PHYTOCHEMICAL ANTIOXIDANTS.

3 to 4 large beets, trimmed
1 tbsp olive oil
1 large onion, chopped
1 tbsp ground cumin
14 oz canned chickpeas, drained
   and rinsed
1 tbsp tahini
⅓ cup low-fat plain yogurt
3 garlic cloves, crushed

¼ cup lemon juice
½ cup reduced-salt vegetable stock
Pita bread, to serve (optional)

PREP TIME: 15 MINUTES
TOTAL COOKING TIME: 40 MINUTES
SERVINGS: 8

Scrub the beets well. Bring a large saucepan of water to a boil and cook the beets for 40 minutes or until soft and cooked through. Drain and cool slightly before peeling.

Meanwhile, heat the oil in a frying pan over medium heat and cook the onion for 2 minutes, or until soft. Add the cumin and cook for a further 1 minute, or until fragrant.

Chop the beets and put in a food processor or blender with the onion mixture, chickpeas, tahini, yogurt, garlic, lemon juice and stock and process until smooth and thoroughly combined. Spoon the hummus into a serving bowl and serve with pita bread.

HINTS:
• This hummus can be a great accompaniment to a main meal or is delicious as part of a meze platter with bruschetta or crusty bread. Its vivid color sparks up any table.
• You can use 1 lb of any vegetable to make the hummus. Try carrot or pumpkin.

nutrition per serving: Energy 116 Cal; Fat 4.8 g; Saturated fat 0.6 g; Protein 4.8 g; Carbohydrate 11.7 g; Fiber 4.1 g; Cholesterol <1 mg; Sodium 184 mg

TABOULEH WITH SOY GRITS

THIS TABOULEH IS A GOOD, GLUTEN-FREE ALTERNATIVE TO REGULAR
TABOULEH. IT IS LOW-GI AND A GOOD SOURCE OF FOLATE.

1 bunch flat-leaf (Italian) parsley
1 cup soy grits
2 tbsp chopped mint
1 small red onion, cut into thin wedges
3 tomatoes, chopped
14 oz canned chickpeas, drained
   and rinsed
3 tbsp lemon juice

2 tbsp extra virgin olive oil
Lebanese or pita bread, to serve (optional)
  (see Hints)

PREP TIME: 20 MINUTES + SOAKING

TOTAL COOKING TIME: NONE

SERVINGS: 6–8

Remove all the parsley leaves from the stalks, roughly chop and put in a large
serving bowl.

Put the soy grits in a heatproof bowl and pour in $2/3$ cup boiling water.
Leave to soak for 3 minutes, or until all the water has been absorbed.

Add the soy grits to the parsley, along with the mint, onion, tomato and chickpeas.
Drizzle with the lemon juice and olive oil. Season well with freshly ground black
pepper and toss together.

Serve with Lebanese or pita bread.

HINTS:
• Soy grits are available from health food shops.
• For a complete gluten-free snack, serve with corn tortillas or gluten-free crackers.

nutrition per serving (8): Energy 224 Cal; Fat 12 g; Saturated fat 1.4 g; Protein 18.1 g; Carbohydrate
9.5 g; Fiber 5.2 g; Cholesterol 0 mg; Sodium 93 mg

SMOKY EGGPLANT TAPENADE

1 large eggplant (about 1 lb)
2 cups pitted kalamata olives
5 anchovy fillets in brine, drained
¼ cup capers, rinsed and squeezed dry
3 garlic cloves, finely chopped
1 small handful flat-leaf (Italian) parsley
1 small handful basil leaves
1 small handful oregano leaves
1 tbsp lemon juice

1 tbsp extra virgin olive oil
crackers or vegetable crudités, to serve
  (optional)

PREP TIME: 20 MINUTES
COOKING TIME: 20 MINUTES
SERVINGS: 10

Preheat the broiler or barbecue grill. Cook the eggplant, turning frequently, for 15–20 minutes, or until the skin is black all over and the flesh is soft. Remove from the heat. When cool enough to handle, cut off the stem, peel off the skin and roughly chop the eggplant flesh.

Put the olives, anchovies, capers, garlic, parsley, basil, oregano, lemon juice and oil in a small processor or blender. Process for 10–15 seconds, or until roughly chopped.

Add the chopped eggplant and blend in 3-second bursts for 15 seconds, or until the tapenade has a medium–smooth consistency with a little texture. Season with freshly ground black pepper and transfer to a serving bowl. Serve with crackers or vegetable crudités.

HINTS:
• Store in an airtight container in the refrigerator for up to a week.
• If you have a gas stove, you can put the eggplant directly on the open flame and follow the same cooking process. This will take half the time and give an even smokier flavor.

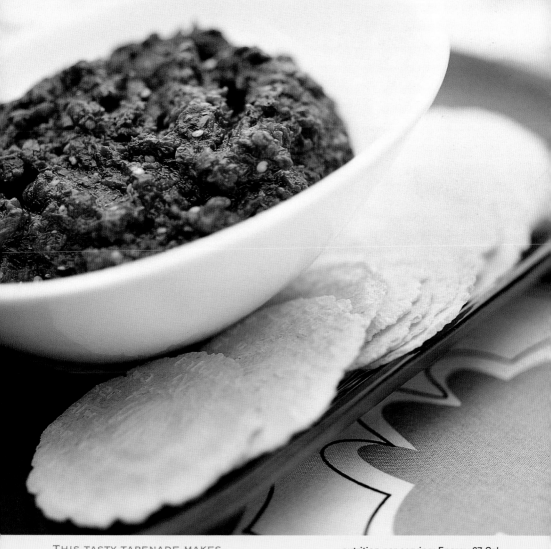

THIS TASTY TAPENADE MAKES
A GREAT DIP FOR PARTIES
OR A SNACK WITH VEGETABLE
CRUDITÉS OR CRACKERS. IT'S
ALSO DELICIOUS AS A SPREAD
ON BREAD INSTEAD OF
MARGARINE.

nutrition per serving: Energy 67 Cal
Fat 2.5 g
Saturated fat 0.4 g
Protein 1.4 g
Carbohydrate 8.8 g
Fiber 1.9 g
Cholesterol 2 mg
Sodium 240 mg

SAN CHOY BAU

THIS TASTY CHINESE FAVORITE IS GREAT TO SERVE AS A STARTER OR LIGHT MEAL WITH FRIENDS. IT'S IMPORTANT TO USE FRESH INGREDIENTS FOR THIS DISH TO ENJOY ITS CRISP, JUICY FLAVORS.

4 dried Chinese mushrooms

3 tsp canola oil, for cooking

¼ cup slivered almonds, chopped

4 oz water chestnuts, drained and finely chopped

1 carrot, finely chopped

4 spring onions (scallions), finely chopped

9 oz lean ground pork

4 cilantro roots, finely chopped

1 tbsp grated fresh ginger

12 lettuce leaves

hoisin sauce, to serve (optional)

SAUCE

1 tbsp reduced-sodium soy sauce

1 tbsp lime juice

1 tsp sesame oil

¼ cup chopped fresh cilantro leaves

2 tbsp chopped fresh mint

PREP TIME: 25 MINUTES +
 10 MINUTES SOAKING

TOTAL COOKING TIME: 10 MINUTES

SERVINGS: 4

Soak the mushrooms in a small bowl of hot water for 10 minutes, or until softened. Discard the tough stems and finely chop the mushroom caps.

To make the sauce, combine the soy sauce, lime juice, sesame oil, cilantro and mint in a small jug.

Heat the wok until very hot, add 1 teaspoon of the oil and swirl around to coat the side. Add the almonds, water chestnuts, carrot and spring onion to the wok and stir-fry for 1 minute, or until they are lightly cooked but not browned—they should still be crisp. Remove from the wok and set aside.

Reheat the wok and add the remaining 2 teaspoons of canola oil. Stir-fry the minced pork, coriander root, ginger and mushrooms over medium–high heat for 2–3 minutes, or until the pork changes color, but do not overcook the pork or it will be tough.

Add the sauce and stir to combine. Return the vegetable mixture to the wok and stir-fry for 1–2 minutes, or until heated through and the mixture is well combined. Spoon the pork mixture into the lettuce leaves and dollop with the hoisin sauce, to taste. Serve more hoisin sauce for dipping.

nutrition per serving: Energy 217 Cal; Fat 13.2 g; Saturated fat 1.8 g; Protein 16 g; Carbohydrate 7.5 g; Fiber 3.7 g; Cholesterol 19 mg; Sodium 253 mg

VIETNAMESE RICE PAPER ROLLS WITH DIPPING SAUCE

THESE FLAVORSOME, REFRESHING RICE PAPER ROLLS ARE LOW IN FAT AND CHOLESTEROL-FREE. THEY ARE GREAT TO SERVE ON A HOT SUMMER DAY.

1¾ oz dried rice vermicelli

7 oz frozen soybeans

16 square 6 in rice paper wrappers

1 zucchini, julienned

1 cucumber, julienned

1 carrot, grated

1 cup mint leaves

3½ oz firm tofu, cut into ½ in strips

DIPPING SAUCE

2 tbsp sweet chili sauce

2 tbsp lime or lemon juice

2 tsp brown sugar

1 tsp reduced-sodium soy sauce or tamari

2 tbsp chopped cilantro leaves

PREPARATION TIME: 40 MINUTES +
    5 MINUTES SOAKING

TOTAL COOKING TIME: 2 MINUTES

SERVINGS: 4

Soak the vermicelli in hot water for 5 minutes, or until soft. Drain and cut into 2 in lengths with a pair of scissors. Bring a saucepan of water to a boil, add the soybeans and cook for 2 minutes. Drain well.

Working with no more than 2 rice paper wrappers at a time, dip each wrapper in a bowl of warm water for 10 seconds to soften. Drain, then lay out on a flat work surface.

Put a small amount of rice vermicelli on the bottom third of a wrapper, leaving a ¾ in border on either side. Top with a little zucchini, cucumber, carrot, soy beans, mint and 2 strips of tofu. Keeping the filling compact and neat, fold in both sides and roll up tightly. Seal with a little water, if necessary. Cover with a damp cloth and repeat with the remaining rice paper wrappers and filling ingredients.

To make the dipping sauce, combine all the ingredients with 2 tablespoons water in a small bowl and stir together well. Serve with the rice paper rolls.

nutrition per serving: Energy 314 Cal; Fat 5.7 g; Saturated fat 0.7 g; Protein 13.5 g; Carbohydrate 49.6 g; Fiber 4.5 g; Cholesterol 0 mg; Sodium 687 mg

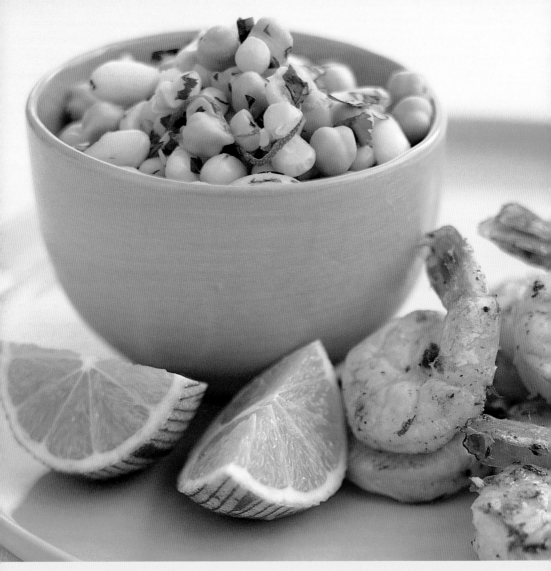

SEAFOOD LOVERS WILL ENJOY THIS
LOW-GI DISH AS A SPECIAL TREAT.
THE SHRIMP PROVIDE IODINE,
PROTEIN AND THE BEANS ARE
RICH IN FIBER.

nutrition per serving: Energy 273 Cal
Fat 7.4 g
Saturated fat 1.1 g
Protein 23.4 g
Carbohydrate 24.8 g
Fiber 8.3 g
Cholesterol 101 mg
Sodium 487 mg

ASIAN-STYLE SHRIMP WITH BEAN AND CORN SALAD

14 oz canned cannellini beans, drained and
  rinsed
10½ oz canned chickpeas, drained
  and rinsed
11 oz canned corn kernels, drained
  and rinsed
1 tsp grated lime zest
2 tbsp chopped cilantro leaves
1 lb raw large shrimp
2 tbsp lemon juice

1 tbsp sesame oil
2 garlic cloves, crushed
2 tsp grated fresh ginger
olive or canola oil spray
lime quarters, to serve

PREP TIME: 10 MINUTES + 3 HOURS
  MARINATING
COOKING TIME: 5 MINUTES
SERVINGS: 4

Combine the cannellini beans, chickpeas and corn kernels in a large bowl. Stir through the lime zest and coriander.

Peel the shrimp, leaving the tails intact. Gently pull out the dark vein from each prawn back, starting at the head end.

To make the marinade, combine the lemon juice, sesame oil, garlic and ginger in a small bowl. Add the shrimp and gently stir to coat them in the marinade. Cover and refrigerate for at least 3 hours.

Heat a castiron skillet until hot. Spray the skillet with oil, then cook the shrimp for 3–5 minutes, or until pink and cooked through. Brush frequently with marinade while cooking. Serve immediately with the bean mixture and wedges of lime.

HINT:
• Alternatively, the shrimp can be threaded onto bamboo skewers. Soak the skewers in cold water for about 30 minutes. This will prevent the skewers burning during cooking. After marinating, thread the shrimp evenly onto the skewers and cook as stated, turning and basting occasionally during cooking.

CHICKPEA FRITTERS

THESE FRITTERS ARE TASTY AND EASY TO EAT, AND WILL BE POPULAR WITH THE WHOLE FAMILY. THEY'RE AN EXCELLENT SOURCE OF FIBER AND ARE FULL OF PROTEIN.

2 tsp olive or canola oil

4 spring onions (scallions), sliced

2 garlic cloves, finely chopped

1 small red chili, seeded and finely chopped

20 oz canned chickpeas, drained and rinsed

2 tbsp chopped cilantro leaves

1 egg, lightly beaten

olive or canola oil spray

99% fat-free tomato salsa, to serve (optional)

mixed-leaf salad, to serve (optional)

PREP TIME: 20 MINUTES

COOKING TIME: 25 MINUTES

MAKES 6

Preheat the oven to 400°F. Line a baking tray with baking paper. Heat the oil in a large non-stick frying pan over medium heat. Add the spring onions, garlic and chili and cook, stirring, for 1–2 minutes, or until the spring onion softens.

Put the chickpeas, spring onion mixture and cilantro in a food processor or blender. Process until the mixture just starts to hold together. Do not overprocess—the mixture should be just roughly processed. Transfer to a bowl and mix in the egg. Using wet hands, shape the mixture into six even fritters.

Lightly spray the fritters with oil and put on prepared tray. Bake for 20 minutes turning once until lightly golden brown. Serve with salsa and a mixed-leaf salad.

nutrition per fritter: Energy 103 Cal; Fat 4.3 g; Saturated fat 0.7 g; Protein 5.5 g; Carbohydrate 9.1 g; Fiber 3.7 g; Cholesterol 31 mg; Sodium 168 mg

HERBED COTTAGE CHEESE POTATO

THIS NOURISHING LIGHT MEAL WILL KEEP YOU GOING. IT'S LOW IN FAT AND PROVIDES GOOD AMOUNTS OF B VITAMINS, BETA-CAROTENE, POTASSIUM AND PHOSPHORUS AS WELL AS CARBOHYDRATE.

4 large russet or sweet potatoes

7 oz blanched, chopped spinach leaves (see Hint)

1 cup low-fat cottage cheese

2 tbsp chopped, mixed herbs (basil, parsley, oregano)

½ cup rinsed, chopped sun-dried tomatoes

4½ oz diced mushrooms

PREP TIME: 20 MINUTES

COOKING TIME: 50 MINUTES

SERVINGS: 4

Preheat the oven to 400°F. Bake the potatoes for 50 minutes, or until cooked through.

Put the spinach leaves, cottage cheese, herbs, sun-dried tomato and mushrooms in a bowl, and mix together well.

Make a deep cut along the top of each cooked potato. Divide the topping among the baked potatoes. Serve hot.

HINT:
• To blanch the spinach, put the spinach leaves in a steamer over boiling water. Blanch for 1 minute then drain well.

nutrition per serving: Energy 262 Cal; Fat 2.6 g; Saturated fat 0.6 g; Protein 18.9 g; Carbohydrate 33.9 g; Fiber 11.2 g; Cholesterol 7 mg; Sodium 164 mg

BAKED SWEET POTATOES WITH AVOCADO AND CORN SALSA

4 medium sweet potatoes
1 red onion, finely chopped
1 avocado, finely chopped
1 tbsp lemon juice
4½ oz canned corn kernels, drained
½ red bell pepper, finely chopped

1 tbsp sweet chili sauce
low-fat plain yogurt, to serve

PREP TIME: 15 MINUTES
COOKING TIME: 50 MINUTES
SERVINGS: 4

Preheat the oven to 400°F. Prick the sweet potatoes a few times with a fork. Bake on an oven rack for 50 minutes, or until cooked through.

Meanwhile, put the onion, avocado, lemon juice, corn and red pepper in a bowl and mix together well. Stir in the chili sauce and season to taste with freshly ground black pepper.

Make a deep cut along the top of each cooked sweet potato. Divide the topping among the sweet potatoes and add a dollop of low-fat plain yogurt.

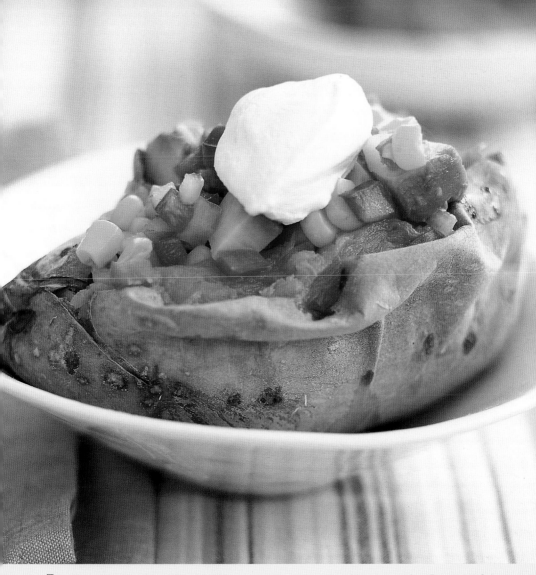

THIS VEGETARIAN BAKED SWEET
POTATO DISH IS A GREAT SOURCE
OF THE ANTIOXIDANTS LUTEIN,
BETA-CAROTENE AND ZEAXANTHIN.
IT'S ALSO LOW IN FAT.

nutrition per serving: Energy 311 Cal
Fat 13.5 g
Saturated fat 2.9 g
Protein 7.3 g
Carbohydrate 37.1 g
Fiber 5.5 g
Cholesterol 1 mg
Sodium 130 mg

SOUPS AND SALADS

JERUSALEM ARTICHOKE SOUP

JERUSALEM ARTICHOKES AREN'T REALLY ARTICHOKES AT ALL, BUT A TYPE OF TUBER. THEY ARE LOW IN CALORIES AND CHOLESTEROL-FREE AND HAVE A SLIGHTLY NUTTY FLAVOR—DELICIOUS IN SOUPS.

1 tbsp olive oil

1 onion, roughly chopped

1 leek, white part only, chopped

1 celery stalk, chopped

2 garlic cloves, chopped

1 lb 12 oz Jerusalem artichokes, cut into 2 in pieces

2 potatoes, cut into 2 in pieces

1 tsp freshly grated nutmeg

1 cup reduced-salt chicken stock or vegetable stock

2 cups low-fat milk

2 tbsps finely snipped chives

PREP TIME: 20 MINUTES

COOKING TIME: 35 MINUTES

SERVINGS: 4

Heat the oil in a large heavy-based saucepan over low heat. Add the onion, leek, celery and garlic and cook for 2 minutes. Cover and simmer, stirring occasionally, for 5 minutes. Do not allow the vegetables to brown.

Add the Jerusalem artichokes, potato and nutmeg and stir to combine. Cook for 2 minutes, then add the stock, 1 cup water and 1 cup of the milk. Bring to a boil, cover and cook for 20 minutes, or until the vegetables are tender.

Remove the saucepan from the heat. Set aside to cool slightly. Using a food processor or blender, process the soup for 10 seconds, or until roughly puréed. Season well with freshly ground black pepper. Stir in the remaining milk and half the chives and gently reheat the soup.

Ladle the soup into four bowls and sprinkle with the remaining chives and some freshly ground black pepper.

HINT:
• The Jerusalem artichokes can be replaced with an equal weight of potatoes. The soup will keep in the refrigerator, covered, for up to 4 days, or in an airtight container in the freezer for up to 1 month.

nutrition per serving: Energy 300 Cal; Fat 5.5 g; Saturated fat 1 g; Protein 14 g; Carbohydrate 43.5 g; Fiber 9.2 g; Cholesterol 6 mg; Sodium 259 mg

SPLIT PEA SOUP

A GREAT WAY TO INCLUDE LEGUMES IN YOUR DIET, THIS NOURISHING SOUP
IS LOW-FAT, LOW-GI AND HIGH IN FIBER.

1 tbsp olive oil

1 large yellow onion, chopped

1 large carrot, cut into ½ in cubes

1 large celery stalk, cut into ½ in cubes

2 bay leaves

1 tbsp finely chopped thyme

6 garlic cloves, finely chopped

2 cups yellow split peas

4 cups reduced-salt chicken stock

¼ cup lemon juice

grainy bread, to serve (optional)

mixed-leaf salad, to serve (optional)

PREP TIME: 20 MINUTES

COOKING TIME: 1 HOUR 30 MINUTES

SERVINGS: 6–8

Heat the oil in a large saucepan over medium heat. Add the onion, carrot and celery, and cook for 4–5 minutes, or until starting to brown. Add the bay leaves, thyme and garlic, and cook for 1 minute.

Stir in the split peas, then add the chicken stock and 4 cups water. Cook for 1 hour 20 minutes, or until the split peas and vegetables are soft. Stir often during cooking to prevent the soup from sticking to the bottom of the pan, and skim any scum from the surface. Add a little extra water if the soup is too thick.

Remove the soup from the heat and discard the bay leaves. Stir in the lemon juice and season with freshly ground black pepper. Serve with grainy bread and a mixed-leaf salad.

nutrition per serving (8): Energy 225 Cal; Fat 3.6 g; Saturated fat 0.5 g; Protein 15.3 g; Carbohydrate 29.7 g; Fiber 6.9 g; Cholesterol 2 mg; Sodium 331 mg

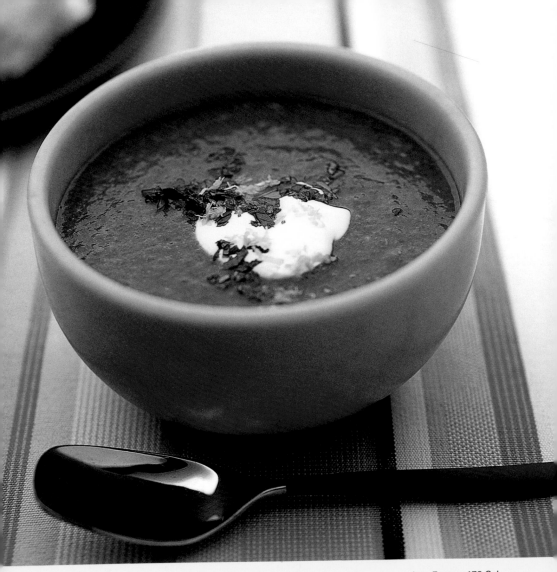

NOTHING SOOTHES LIKE A
WARM BOWL OF SOUP ON
A COLD WINTER NIGHT. THIS
FRENCH CLASSIC IS SURE TO
MAKE YOU FEEL SATISFIED.

nutrition per serving: Energy 173 Cal
Fat 8 g
Saturated fat 2.5 g
Protein 8.5 g
Carbohydrate 14.3 g
Fiber 4.5 g
Cholesterol 3 mg
Sodium 359 mg

ALSACE MUSHROOM SOUP

¼ oz dried porcini mushrooms

1 tbsp olive oil

1 onion, roughly chopped

4 French shallots, chopped

1 large potato, chopped

1 celery stalk, chopped

2 garlic cloves, chopped

1 small red chilli, seeded and chopped

6 oz flat mushrooms, roughly chopped

6 oz Swiss brown mushrooms, roughly chopped

2 cups reduced-salt chicken stock or vegetable stock

2 large thyme sprigs

1–2 tsp lemon juice, to taste

⅓ cup extra-light sour cream, to serve

2 tbsp finely chopped flat-leaf (Italian) parsley, to serve

1 tbsp grated lemon zest, to serve

PREP TIME: 25 MINUTES + 10 MINUTES SOAKING

COOKING TIME: 30 MINUTES

SERVINGS: 4

Put the porcini mushrooms in a small bowl and pour 1 cup hot water over them. Set aside to soften for 10 minutes.

Meanwhile, heat the oil in a large heavy-based saucepan. Add the onion, shallots, potato, celery, garlic and chilli. Stir for 2 minutes to coat the vegetables in the margarine. Reduce the heat, cover and simmer, stirring occasionally, for 5 minutes. Do not allow the vegetables to brown.

Add the fresh mushrooms to the saucepan and cook, stirring, for 2–3 minutes. Add the stock, 1 cup water, thyme sprigs and porcini mushrooms with their soaking water. Slowly bring to a boil over low heat, then reduce the heat and simmer, covered, for 15 minutes. Discard the thyme sprigs. Set aside to cool slightly.

Using a food processor or blender, process the soup for 15–20 seconds, or until roughly puréed. The soup should still have texture. Add the lemon juice, to taste, and season well with freshly ground black pepper. Gently reheat the soup and ladle into warm bowls. Top with a spoonful of the sour cream and sprinkle with the parsley and lemon zest.

HINT:

- The soup will keep in the refrigerator, covered, for up to 4 days, or in an airtight container in the freezer for up to 1 month.

SCOTCH BROTH

BARLEY IS A GOOD GRAIN TO INCLUDE IN YOUR DIET IF YOU ARE TRYING TO LOWER YOUR CHOLESTEROL—IT'S LOW-GI AND A GOOD SOURCE OF SOLUBLE FIBER. THIS BROTH ALSO CONTAINS B-GROUP VITAMINS, IRON AND ZINC.

2 to 2½ lb lamb shanks, cut in half through the bone (ask your butcher to do this)
3 onions, chopped
3 turnips, chopped
2 carrots, chopped
1 tbsp black peppercorns
½ cup pearl barley
1 carrot, diced, extra
2 onions, finely chopped, extra
2 turnips, diced, extra

1 leek, white part only, chopped
1 celery stalk, diced
chopped flat-leaf (Italian) parsley, to serve

PREP TIME: 40 MINUTES + 1 HOUR SOAKING + OVERNIGHT REFRIGERATION
COOKING TIME: 3 HOURS 35 MINUTES
SERVINGS: 8

To make the stock, put the lamb shanks, onion, turnip, carrot, peppercorns and 8 cups water in a large saucepan. Bring to a boil, reduce the heat and simmer, covered, for 3 hours. Skim the surface as required.

Remove the shanks and any meat that has fallen off the bones and cool slightly. Remove the meat from the bones and finely chop, then cover and refrigerate. Strain the stock, discarding the vegetables. Cool the stock and refrigerate overnight, or until the fat has set on top and can be spooned off. Cover the barley with water and soak for 1 hour, then drain.

Put the stock in a large pan and gently reheat. Add the barley, extra carrot, onion and turnip, and the leek and celery. Bring to a boil, reduce the heat and simmer for 30 minutes, or until the barley and vegetables are just cooked. Return the meat to the pan and simmer for 5 minutes. Season well with freshly ground black pepper and serve with the parsley.

nutrition per serving: Energy 228 Cal; Fat 6.7 g; Saturated fat 3.3 g; Protein 22.5 g; Carbohydrate 16.3 g; Fiber 5.7 g; Cholesterol 65 mg; Sodium 91 mg

BEET AND RED PEPPER SOUP

THIS COLOURFUL SOUP WITH THE GOODNESS OF BEETS AND BELL PEPPERS
IS LOW IN FAT AND A RICH SOURCE OF THE ANTIOXIDANT BETA-CAROTENE.

**6 beets, about 1 lb without stems and
  leaves**
1 tbsp olive oil
1 red onion, chopped
1 celery stalk, chopped
1 garlic clove, chopped
1 large red pepper, chopped
15 oz can reduced-salt diced tomatoes
1 tbsp red wine vinegar

**extra-light sour cream or low-fat plain
  yogurt, to serve (optional)**
2 tbsp finely snipped chives, to serve

PREP TIME: 20 MINUTES
COOKING TIME: 50 MINUTES
SERVINGS: 4

Peel the beets with a vegetable peeler and cut them into 1¼ in cubes. Put the beets in a large saucepan with 4 cups water. Slowly bring to a boil over low to medium heat, then reduce the heat and simmer for 25–30 minutes, or until the beets are tender when pierced with a fork. Remove about ½ cup of beetroot cubes, dice finely and set aside.

Meanwhile, heat the oil in a large heavy-based saucepan over medium heat. Add the onion, celery, garlic and red pepper and stir to coat the vegetables in the oil. Reduce the heat to low, cover and cook, stirring occasionally, for 10 minutes. Do not allow the vegetables to brown. Add the chopped tomatoes and vinegar and simmer for 10 minutes.

Transfer the tomato mixture to the saucepan containing the beets and remove the pan from the heat. Set aside to cool slightly. Using a food processor or blender, process the soup for 20–30 seconds, or until smooth. Season well with freshly ground black pepper.

Ladle the soup into four warm bowls and top with a spoonful of sour cream, the reserved diced beetroot and the chives.

HINT:
• The soup will keep in the refrigerator, covered, for up to 4 days, or in an airtight container in the freezer for up to 1 month.

nutrition per serving: Energy 144 Cal; Fat 5 g; Saturated fat 0.6 g; Protein 4.3 g; Carbohydrate 17.4 g; Fiber 5.5 g; Cholesterol 0 mg; Sodium 99 mg

SPICED PUMPKIN AND LENTIL SOUP

1 tbsp olive oil
1 large onion, chopped
3 garlic cloves, chopped
1 tsp ground turmeric
½ tsp ground coriander
½ tsp ground cumin
½ tsp chilli flakes
4½ cups pumpkin or winter squash, chopped

½ cup canned red lentils, drained and rinsed
⅓ cup plain low-fat yogurt, to serve

PREP TIME: 20 MINUTES
COOKING TIME: 30 MINUTES
SERVINGS: 4

Heat the oil in a large saucepan over medium heat. Add the onion and garlic and fry for 5 minutes, or until softened, being careful not to burn the garlic. Add the turmeric, coriander, cumin and chilli flakes and fry, stirring constantly, for 2 minutes.

Add the pumpkin, red lentils and 4 cups boiling water. Bring to a boil, then reduce the heat and simmer, covered, for 20 minutes, or until the pumpkin and lentils are tender. Set aside to cool for 5 minutes.

Using a food processor or blender, process the soup for 25–35 seconds, or until evenly chopped. Season well with freshly ground black pepper and reheat the soup.

Ladle the soup into four bowls, top with a spoonful of the yogurt and sprinkle with more pepper.

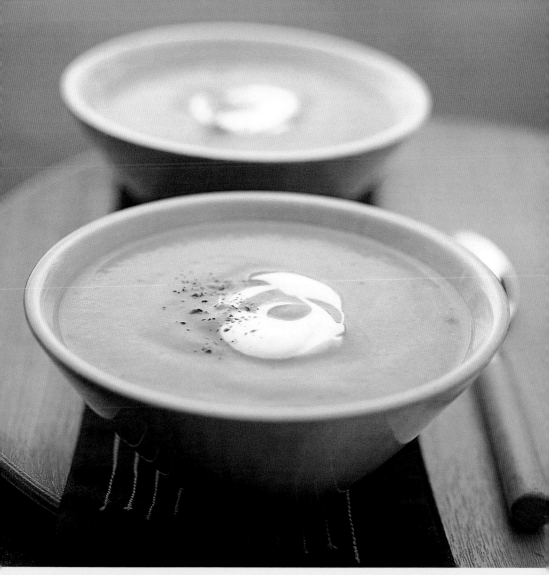

THIS IS A NUTRITIOUS AND
SATISFYING SOUP THAT IS SURE
TO MAKE YOU FEEL FULL.
THE ADDITION OF LENTILS
MAKES IT MORE NUTRITIOUS
AND LOWER GI THAN REGULAR
PUMPKIN SOUP.

nutrition per serving: Energy 233 Cal
Fat 6.2 g
Saturated fat 1.3 g
Protein 13.5 g
Carbohydrate 27.6 g
Fiber 7.7 g
Cholesterol 1 mg
Sodium 28 mg

77

COUSCOUS SALAD

THIS SALAD IS A GOOD CHOICE FOR ACTIVE PEOPLE. IT'S LOW IN FAT AND HIGH IN CARBOHYDRATE AND PROVIDES GOOD AMOUNTS OF FIBER, BETA-CAROTENE AND B-GROUP VITAMINS.

1 large sweet potato, cubed
1 cup green beans, halved
2 cups instant couscous
2 cups boiling reduced-salt chicken stock
7 oz cherry tomatoes, halved
1 cup frozen corn kernels, thawed
1 cup frozen peas, thawed
1 red pepper, chopped
1 cup chopped parsley
½ cup chopped mint

DRESSING
1 garlic clove, crushed
2 tbsp lemon juice
1 tbsp olive oil
1 tsp honey
½ tsp grainy mustard

PREP TIME: 20 MINUTES + 5 MINUTES
    STANDING
COOKING TIME: 15 MINUTES
SERVINGS: 6

Boil or steam the sweet potato and beans in separate saucepans until tender, then drain. Put the couscous in a large bowl and pour on a boiling stock. Cover and leave for 5 minutes, or until all the liquid has been absorbed. Fluff with a fork to separate the grains.

Add the sweet potato, beans, tomato, corn, peas, red pepper and herbs to the couscous, and mix together well.

Put the garlic, lemon juice, oil, honey and mustard in a bowl, and whisk together. Pour the dressing over the salad and toss well.

nutrition per serving: Energy 355 Cal; Fat 4.1 g; Saturated fat 0.6 g; Protein 13.3 g; Carbohydrate 62.4 g; Fiber 5.9 g; Cholesterol 2 mg; Sodium 234 mg

CHICKPEA AND ROAST VEGETABLE SALAD

THIS HEALTHY SALAD IS AN EASY WAY TO EAT LEGUMES AND VEGETABLES.
IT IS LOW IN FAT AND RICH IN BETA-CAROTENE AND SOLUBLE FIBER.

1 large (about 1 lb) butternut squash,
   cubed
2 red red peppers, halved
4 slender eggplants, cut in half lengthways
4 zucchini, cut in half lengthways
4 onions, quartered
olive oil spray
20 oz canned chickpeas, drained
   and rinsed
2 tbsp chopped fresh flat-leaf (Italian)
   parsley

DRESSING
3 tbsp lemon juice
2 tbsp olive oil
1 garlic clove, crushed
1 tsp finely chopped thyme

PREP TIME: 25 MINUTES +
   30 MINUTES STANDING
TOTAL COOKING TIME: 40 MINUTES
SERVINGS: 8

Preheat the oven to 425°F. Line 2 baking trays with baking paper and lay out the vegetables in a single layer and spray them with oil.

Bake for 40 minutes, or until the vegetables are tender and begin to brown slightly on the edges. Cool. Remove the skins from the red pepper if you want. Chop the pepper, eggplant and zucchini into pieces, then put the vegetables in a bowl with the chickpeas and half the parsley.

Whisk together all the dressing ingredients. Season with freshly ground black pepper, then toss with the vegetables. Leave for 30 minutes, then sprinkle with the rest of the parsley.

nutrition per serving: Energy 158 Cal; Fat 6.8 g; Saturated fat 1.1 g; Protein 6.2 g; Carbohydrate 15.6 g; Fiber 5.3 g; Cholesterol 0 mg; Sodium 122 mg

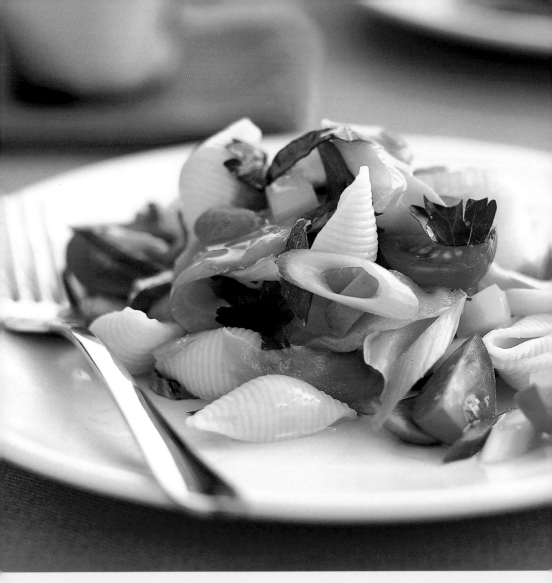

THIS LOW-GI SALAD IS QUICK AND
EASY TO PREPARE FOR LUNCH OR
DINNER. IT CONTAINS SOME
ESSENTIAL OMEGA-3 FATTY ACIDS
AND GOOD AMOUNTS OF
POTASSIUM, ANTIOXIDANTS,
FOLATE AND PHOSPHORUS.

nutrition per serving (6): Energy 324 Cal
Fat 5.5 g
Saturated fat 0.9 g
Protein 16 g
Carbohydrate 50.1 g
Fiber 3.7 g
Cholesterol 16 mg
Sodium 574 mg

HERBED PASTA AND SALMON SALAD

14 oz small pasta shells

9 oz cherry tomatoes, quartered,
    or halved, if small

1 large yellow red pepper, seeded and
    diced

2 celery stalks, thinly sliced

3 spring onions (scallions), thinly sliced

¼ cup pitted green olives in brine, drained
    and chopped

2 tbsp capers, rinsed and chopped
    (optional)

7 oz smoked salmon, sliced

1 handful basil, finely shredded

3 tbsp finely chopped flat-leaf (Italian)
    parsley

DRESSING

1 tbsp olive oil

1½ tbsps white wine vinegar

½ tsp dijon mustard

1 tsp honey

PREP TIME: 15 MINUTES

COOKING TIME: 10 MINUTES

SERVINGS: 4–6

Cook the pasta in a large saucepan of boiling water for 10 minutes, or until *al dente*. Rinse under cold water to cool. Drain. Put in a large bowl.

To make the dressing, whisk all the ingredients together. Put all the other ingredients into the bowl with the pasta, add the dressing and toss together. Season with freshly ground black pepper and serve.

HINT:
• Any type of small pasta shapes can be used in this recipe.

81

TUNA AND BEAN SALAD

BASED ON FISH AND BEANS, THIS SALAD CONTAINS FILLING PROTEIN, LOW-GI
CARBOHYDRATE AND FIBER, PLUS GOOD AMOUNTS OF B-GROUP VITAMINS,
VITAMIN C, POTASSIUM AND HEART-HEALTHY OMEGA-3 FATTY ACIDS.

3½ oz green beans, chopped
1 cup frozen lima beans, thawed
15 oz canned tuna in spring water, drained
7 oz cherry tomatoes, quartered
1 red onion, thinly sliced
3½ oz mixed salad leaves
3½ oz arugula leaves

DRESSING
1 tbsp extra virgin olive oil
2 tbsp lemon juice
1 tsp honey
1 garlic clove, crushed
2 tbsp chopped dill

PREP TIME: 20 MINUTES + 10 MINUTES
REFRIGERATION
COOKING TIME: 5 MINUTES
SERVINGS: 4

Steam the green beans until tender, rinse under cold water and drain. Put the green and lima beans, tuna, tomato and onion in a bowl, and toss well.

To make the dressing, whisk all the ingredients together. Pour the dressing over the tuna mixture, cover and refrigerate for 10 minutes.

Combine the salad leaves and arugula, and arrange on a salad platter. Top with the tuna mixture and serve.

nutrition per serving: Energy 235 Cal; Fat 7.1 g; Saturated fat 1.4 g; Protein 25.6 g; Carbohydrate 14.1 g; Fiber 7 g; Cholesterol 39 mg; Sodium 85 mg

COLD CHICKEN AND MANGO SALAD WITH HONEY DRESSING

This tangy salad is bursting with flavor. It is very easy to make, completely satisfying and low in fat.

DRESSING
2 tbsp rice vinegar
3 tsp honey
1¼ in piece ginger, chopped
1 tbsp canola oil
1 tsp sesame oil

4½ oz mixed Asian salad leaves
1 large mango, thinly sliced
1 cup yellow or red cherry tomatoes, halved

½ small red onion, sliced into thin wedges
1 cold barbecued chicken, fat and skin removed, meat shredded
¾ cup snow pea sprouts, trimmed
2 tsp toasted sesame seeds

PREP TIME: 15 MINUTES

COOKING TIME: NONE

SERVINGS: 4

To make the dressing, put the vinegar, honey and ginger in a mini food processor or blender and process in 3-second bursts for 20 seconds, or until finely chopped. With the motor running, slowly pour in the oils and blend for 20 seconds, or until thick and creamy.

Arrange the salad leaves on individual plates and top with the mango, tomatoes, onion, chicken and snow pea sprouts. Drizzle with the dressing and sprinkle with the sesame seeds. Serve immediately.

nutrition per serving: Energy 352 Cal; Fat 16.7 g; Saturated fat 3.4 g; Protein 33.4 g; Carbohydrate 15.9 g; Fiber 2.5 g; Cholesterol 114 mg; Sodium 115 mg

PESTO BEEF SALAD

1 large red red pepper
1 large yellow pepper
olive or canola oil spray
3½ oz lean beef fillet steak, trimmed
4½ oz penne pasta
3½ oz button mushrooms, quartered

PESTO
½ bunch basil (about 1¾ oz leaves)
2 garlic cloves, chopped
2 tbsp pumpkin seeds
1 tbsp olive oil
2 tbsp orange juice
1 tbsp lemon juice

PREP TIME: 30 MINUTES + 5 MINUTES
   STANDING
COOKING TIME: 25 MINUTES
SERVINGS: 4

Cut the peppers into large flat pieces, removing the seeds and membrane. Put, skin side up, under a hot broiler until blackened. Leave covered with a dish towel until cool, then peel away the skin and chop the flesh.

Heat a frying pan over medium heat and spray with oil, then cook the steak over high heat for 3–4 minutes on each side. Remove and leave for 5 minutes before cutting into thin slices.

To make the pesto, finely chop the basil leaves, garlic and pumpkin seeds in a food processor. With the motor running, add the oil, orange and lemon juice. Season well with freshly ground black pepper.

Meanwhile, cook the pasta in a large saucepan of boiling water for 10 minutes, or until *al dente*. Drain well and toss with the pesto in a large bowl.

Add the red pepper pieces, steak slices and mushroom quarters to the penne and toss to distribute evenly. Serve immediately.

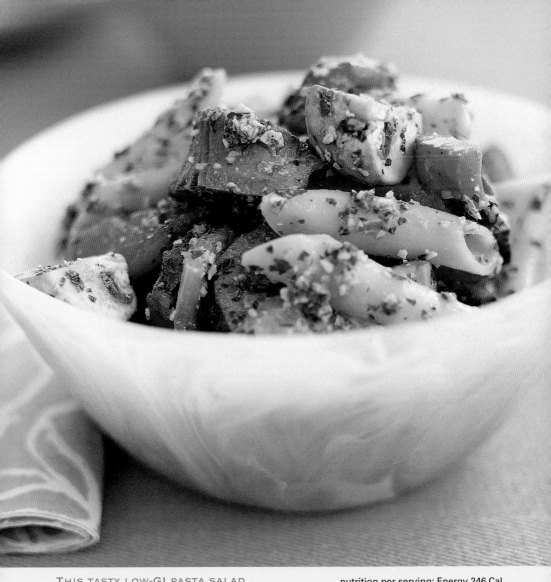

THIS TASTY LOW-GI PASTA SALAD
IS A GREAT CHOICE FOR PEOPLE
WHO NEED TO EAT MORE IRON.
THE PESTO IN THIS DISH IS MUCH
LOWER IN FAT THAN REGULAR
PESTO, AND THE DISH PROVIDES
GOOD AMOUNTS OF ANTIOXIDANTS,
VITAMIN C AND BETA-CAROTENE.

nutrition per serving: Energy 246 Cal
Fat 9.5 g
Saturated fat 1.7 g
Protein 12.3 g
Carbohydrate 25.7 g
Fiber 3.6 g
Cholesterol 17 mg
Sodium 20 mg

TANDOORI LAMB SALAD

THIS INDIAN-STYLE SALAD IS HIGH IN PROTEIN AND A GOOD SOURCE OF IRON, ZINC, POTASSIUM, PHOSPHORUS, FOLATE, NIACIN AND BETA-CAROTENE.

1 cup low-fat plain yogurt
2 garlic cloves, crushed
2 tsp grated fresh ginger
2 tsp ground turmeric
2 tsp ground garam masala
¼ tsp paprika
2 tsp ground coriander
1 lb lean lamb fillets
4 tbsp lemon juice
1½ tsp chopped coriander leaves

1 tsp chopped mint
5 oz mixed salad leaves
1 large mango, cut into strips
2 cucumbers, julienned

PREP TIME: 20 MINUTES + OVERNIGHT
   MARINATING
TOTAL COOKING TIME: 15 MINUTES
SERVINGS: 4

Mix the yogurt, garlic, ginger, dried herbs and spices in a bowl and toss with the lamb to thoroughly coat. Cover and refrigerate overnight.

Broil the lamb on a foil-lined baking tray under high heat for 7 minutes each side, or until the marinade starts to brown. Set aside for 5 minutes before serving.

Mix the lemon juice, coriander and mint then season with freshly ground black pepper. Toss with the salad leaves, mango and cucumber, then arrange on plates. Slice the lamb and serve over the salad.

nutrition per serving: Energy 244 Cal; Fat 5.4 g; Saturated fat 2.1 g; Protein 31.4 g; Carbohydrate 14.5 g; Fiber 3.5 g; Cholesterol 84 mg; Sodium 144 mg

VIETNAMESE RICE NOODLE SALAD

THIS FRESH, ZESTY VIETNAMESE CLASSIC IS A GOOD CHOICE ON A HOT
SUMMER DAY. IT PROVIDES ANTIOXIDANTS AND MINERALS.

7 oz dried vermicelli
½ cup crushed roasted peanuts
½ cup Vietnamese mint, torn
½ cup cilantro leaves
½ red onion, cut into thin wedges
1 green mango, julienned
1 cucumber, halved lengthways and thinly
  sliced diagonally

LEMON GRASS DRESSING
½ cup lime juice
1 tbsp shaved palm sugar or brown sugar
3 tbsp seasoned rice vinegar
2 lemon grass stems, finely chopped
3 kaffir lime leaves, finely shredded

PREP TIME: 20 MINUTES + 10 MINUTES
  STANDING + 30 MINUTES REFRIGERATION
TOTAL COOKING TIME: NONE
SERVINGS: 4–6

Put the rice vermicelli in a bowl and cover with boiling water. Leave for 10 minutes or until soft, then drain, rinse under cold water and cut into short lengths.

Put the vermicelli, peanuts, mint, cilantro, onion, mango and cucumber in a large bowl and toss together.

To make the dressing, put all the ingredients in a jar with a lid and shake.

Toss the salad and dressing and refrigerate for 30 minutes before serving.

nutrition per serving (6): Energy 236 Cal; Fat 6.7 g; Saturated fat 0.8 g; Protein 6.8 g; Carbohydrate 35.5 g; Fiber 2.6 g; Cholesterol 0 mg; Sodium 9 mg

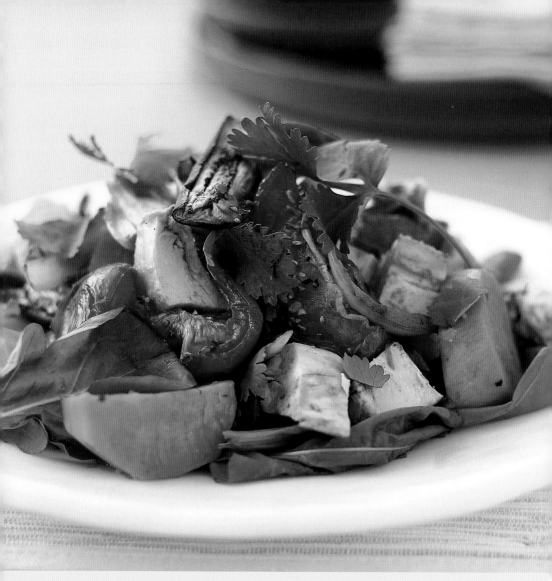

ADDING A VARIETY OF HEALTHY
INGREDIENTS FROM DIFFERENT
FOOD GROUPS MAKES A SALAD
MORE SATISFYING AND NUTRITIOUS,
AND HELPS YOU MEET HEALTHY
EATING GUIDELINES. THIS SALAD
FITS THE BILL!

nutrition per serving: Energy 236 Cal
Fat 7.7 g
Saturated fat 2 g
Protein 23.9 g
Carbohydrate 15.7 g
Fiber 3.7 g
Cholesterol 76 mg
Sodium 150 mg

CHICKEN AND SWEET POTATO SALAD

4 roma (plum) tomatoes, quartered
  lengthways
1 large eggplant, quartered lengthways
olive oil spray
2 large sweet potatoes, cut into ¾ in slices
1 large red onion, sliced into thin wedges
1 barbecued chicken
2 tbsp chopped cilantro leaves

2–3 tbsp balsamic vinegar
2 handfuls arugula

PREP TIME: 30 MINUTES
COOKING TIME: 50 MINUTES
SERVINGS: 6

Preheat the oven to 400°F. Put the tomatoes and eggplant on a large, non-stick baking tray, spray with a little oil and season with freshly ground black pepper. Bake, turning the eggplant halfway through, for 25–30 minutes.

Meanwhile, steam the sweet potato for 15 minutes, or until just tender. Put in a large bowl with the tomato and eggplant.

Lightly spray a small non-stick frying pan with oil, add the onion and cook over low heat for 6 minutes, or until golden. Set aside.

Remove the skin and bones from the chicken and discard. Cut the chicken meat into bite-sized pieces and add to the vegetables with the cilantro and 1 tablespoon balsamic vinegar. Toss gently.

Put the arugula on a platter, then the chicken mixture and top with the onion. Drizzle with the remaining balsamic vinegar to taste. Serve with thick slices of wholegrain bread.

HINT:
• You can substitute the barbecued chicken with freshly-cooked chicken breast fillets or you can use precooked chicken breast meat, which you'll find in the meat section of the supermarket.

MAIN MEALS

CHICKEN CACCIATORE

THIS LOW-FAT VERSION OF A POPULAR ITALIAN DISH PROVIDES PROTEIN, MONOUNSATURATED FAT, POTASSIUM, NIACIN AND ANTIOXIDANTS.

1 lb lean chicken breast fillets
all-purpose flour, for dusting
2 tsp olive oil
2 onions, thinly sliced
2 garlic cloves, finely chopped
2 anchovy fillets in brine, drained and
   chopped
15 oz can reduced-salt diced tomatoes
½ cup dry white wine
3 tbsp no-added-salt tomato paste
1 tsp brown sugar

6 Kalamata olives, pitted and chopped
chopped fresh flat-leaf (Italian) parsley,
   to garnish
fusilli pasta or boiled potatoes, to serve
   (optional)

PREP TIME: 25 MINUTES
COOKING TIME: 40 MINUTES
SERVINGS: 4

Trim any fat from the chicken and lightly dust the fillets with flour. Heat the oil in a large, heavy-based non-stick frying pan and cook the chicken over high heat for 10 minutes, turning until golden and almost cooked. (If the chicken begins to stick, sprinkle with water and reduce the heat.) Remove, drain on paper towels, cover and set aside.

Add the onion to the pan with the garlic, anchovies and 1 tablespoon water. Cover and cook for 5 minutes, stirring. Add the tomato, wine, tomato paste, sugar and 1 scant cup water. Bring to a boil, then reduce the heat and simmer for 20 minutes. Season with freshly ground black pepper.

Return the chicken and juices to the pan. Add the olives and simmer for 5 minutes, or until the chicken is heated through. Garnish with parsley. Serve with fusilli pasta or boiled potatoes.

nutrition per serving: Energy 254 Cal; Fat 4.5 g; Saturated fat 1.1 g; Protein 30.8 g; Carbohydrate 15.2 g; Fiber 3.3 g; Cholesterol 83 mg; Sodium 203 mg

CORAL TROUT WITH GARLIC TOMATOES AND GREMOLATA

STRONG FLAVORS ABOUND IN THIS TASTY, LOW-FAT DISH. IT IS QUICK TO PREPARE AND IS A GOOD SOURCE OF PROTEIN, BETA-CAROTENE AND OTHER ANTIOXIDANTS.

8 vine-ripened tomatoes, halved

12 garlic cloves, unpeeled

2 tbsp balsamic vinegar

1 tbsp brown sugar

olive or canola oil spray

1½ to 2 lb new potatoes

10½ oz asparagus, trimmed

7 oz coral trout fillets or firm white fish fillets

GREMOLATA

3 handfuls flat-leaf (Italian) parsley, finely chopped

2 tsp lemon zest

2 garlic cloves, finely chopped

PREP TIME: 20 MINUTES

COOKING TIME: 55 MINUTES

SERVINGS: 4

Preheat the oven to 400°F. Line a large baking tray with baking paper. Put the tomatoes, cut-side-up, on the prepared tray. Scatter around the garlic cloves. Pour over the combined balsamic vinegar and sugar. Spray lightly with the oil. Bake the tomatoes and garlic for 30 minutes, or until softened. Remove the garlic after 15 minutes and baste the tomatoes with the balsamic vinegar and sugar. Squeeze out the soft garlic from the cloves and add to the mushy tomatoes.

Combine the gremolata ingredients in a small bowl.

Bring a large saucepan of water to a boil. Cook the potatoes for 12 minutes, or until cooked when tested with a skewer. Drain. Steam the asparagus for 3–4 minutes, or until just tender.

Pat the fish dry with paper towels. Spray a large, non-stick frying pan with oil and lightly spray the fish. Cook the fish for 3–4 minutes on each side, or until browned on both sides and just cooked through.

To serve, pile the tomato and garlic onto serving plates. Top with the fish fillets and spoon over some gremolata. Serve with a boiled new potatoes and steamed asparagus to the side.

nutrition per serving: Energy 420 Cal; Fat 5.3 g; Saturated fat 1.3 g; Protein 48.7 g; Carbohydrate 36.3 g; Fiber 10.9 g; Cholesterol 96 mg; Sodium 169 mg

BLUE-EYE COD IN CHERMOULA

CHERMOULA
1½ tbsp cumin seeds
2 tsp coriander seeds
1 tbsp sweet paprika
pinch cayenne pepper
2 large handfuls cilantro, chopped
1 large handful flat-leaf (Italian) parsley,
  chopped
4 large garlic cloves, crushed
2 tbsp olive oil
4 tbsp lemon juice

6 oz blue-eye cod steaks or other firm
  white fish steaks
1 ½ lb small new potatoes
2 large zucchinis, thickly sliced
4 oz can baby corn

PREP TIME: 20 MINUTES + 1 HOUR
  MARINATING
COOKING TIME: 20 MINUTES
SERVINGS: 4

To make the chermoula, place the cumin and coriander seeds, paprika and cayenne pepper in a small, dry frying pan and toast for 1 minute over medium heat, or until fragrant. Put in a spice grinder, or use a mortar and pestle, and grind to a fine powder. Put in a food processor with the coriander, parsley, garlic, oil and lemon juice. Season with freshly ground black pepper and process until well combined.

Put the fish in a flat, non-metallic dish and pour over the chermoula. Toss to coat well, cover and marinate in the refrigerator for 1 hour.

Bring a large saucepan of water to a boil and cook the potatoes for 10–12 minutes, or until cooked when tested with a skewer. Steam the zucchini and corn for 3 minutes, or until just cooked.

Meanwhile, remove the fish from the chermoula, reserving the liquid. Heat a chargrill plate or barbecue over a high heat and cook the fish for 2–3 minutes on each side, basting with the remaining chermoula. Serve immediately with the potatoes, zucchini and corn.

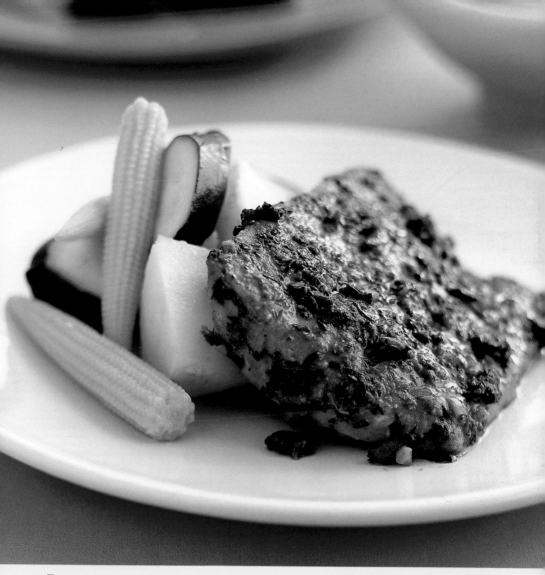

THIS LOW-FAT DISH IS A GOOD
CHOICE IF YOU'RE WATCHING
YOUR WEIGHT AS IT CONTAINS
HIGHLY FILLING FISH PROTEIN.

nutrition per serving: Energy 396 Cal
Fat 12.1 g
Saturated fat 1.6 g
Protein 34.4 g
Carbohydrate 31.9 g
Fiber 8.9 g
Cholesterol 78 mg
Sodium 151 mg

FISH TIKKA

WHY ORDER INDIAN TAKEOUT WHEN YOU CAN MAKE YOUR OWN? THIS TASTY
DISH IS EASY TO EAT AND SURE TO PLEASE THE WHOLE FAMILY.

MARINADE

1 cup low-fat plain yogurt

2 spring onions (scallions), finely chopped

1 tbsp grated fresh ginger

2 garlic cloves, crushed

2 tbsp lemon juice

1 tsp ground coriander

1 tbsp garam masala

1 tsp paprika

1 tsp chilli powder

2 tbsp no-added-salt tomato paste

1 lb skinless firm white fish fillets (such as
    flake, sea bream, snapper, grouper or
    orange roughy)

2 onions, each cut into 8 chunks

2 small green or red peppers, each cut into
    8 chunks

boiled rice, to serve (optional)

lemon wedges, to serve

YOGURT DRESSING

about 1/3 cup peeled, diced cucumber

1 tbsp chopped cilantro leaves

1 cup low-fat plain yogurt

PREP TIME: 25 MINUTES +
    1 HOUR MARINATING

COOKING TIME: 6 MINUTES

SERVINGS: 4

Mix all the marinade ingredients together in a shallow non-metallic dish long enough and
deep enough to hold eight long metal skewers.

Cut the fish into 24 bite-sized chunks. On each skewer, thread 3 fish pieces, 2 onion
pieces and 2 pepper pieces, alternating them as you go. Turn the skewers about in the
marinade so that all the fish and vegetables are well coated. Cover and marinate in the
refrigerator for at least 1 hour, or overnight if convenient.

Mix the yogurt dressing ingredients together in a small bowl and set aside.

Heat the barbecue or broiler to its highest setting. When the barbecue or broiler is very
hot, lift the skewers out of the marinade and grill for 5–6 minutes, or until the fish is firm
and slightly charred. Serve with the yogurt dressing and lemon wedges.

nutrition per serving: Energy 280 Cal; Fat 9; g; Saturated fat 4.3 g; Protein 33.2 g; Carbohydrate 13.4
g; Fiber 3 g; Cholesterol 104 mg; Sodium 263 mg

BARBECUED PORK AND BROCCOLI

A CHINESE STREET-STALL CLASSIC CAN BE A HIT IN YOUR HOME TOO WITH
THIS TASTY RECIPE.

2 tsp canola oil
1 large onion, thinly sliced
2 carrots, julienned
1 bunch broccoli, chopped
6 spring onions (scallions), diagonally
  sliced
1 tbsp finely chopped fresh ginger
3 garlic cloves, finely chopped
1 lb Chinese barbecued pork, thinly sliced
  and trimmed of fat

1 tbsp reduced-sodium soy sauce
2 tbsp mirin
2 cups bean sprouts
boiled basmati rice, to serve (optional)

PREP TIME: 25 MINUTES
TOTAL COOKING TIME: 10 MINUTES
SERVINGS: 4

Heat a wok until very hot, add the oil and swirl it around to coat the side. Stir-fry the onion
over medium heat for 3–4 minutes, or until slightly softened. Add the carrot, broccoli, spring
onion, ginger and garlic and cook for 4–5 minutes, tossing the mixture constantly.

Increase the heat to high and add the barbecued pork. Toss constantly until the pork is
well mixed with the vegetables and is heated through. Add the soy sauce and mirin, and
toss until the ingredients are well coated. (The wok should be hot enough for the sauce to
reduce into a glaze.) Add the bean sprouts and season with freshly ground black pepper.
Serve immediately with a boiled rice.

HINT:
• Barbecued pork is available from Asian food stores.

nutrition per serving: Energy 463 Cal; Fat 6.6; g; Saturated fat 1.5 g; Protein 28.6 g; Carbohydrate
65.4 g; Fiber 7.3 g; Cholesterol 54 mg; Sodium 546 mg

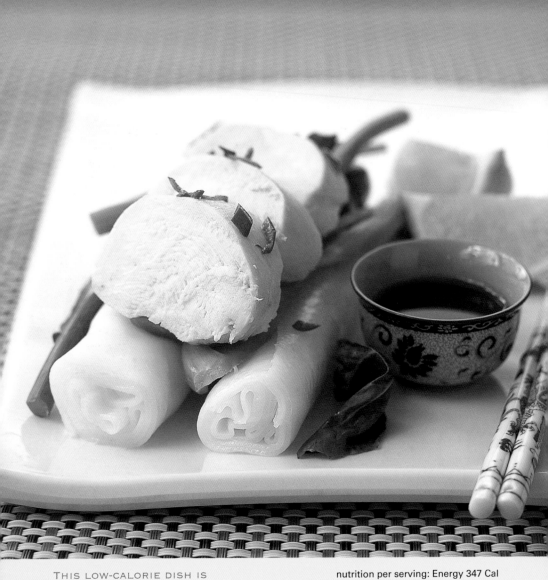

THIS LOW-CALORIE DISH IS
HIGH IN VITAMINS A AND C,
CALCIUM AND PROTEIN.

nutrition per serving: Energy 347 Cal

Fat 5.0 g

Saturated fat 1.2 g

Protein 38.0 g

Carbohydrate 35.2 g

Fiber 3.8 g

Cholesterol 97 g

Sodium 293 mg

LEMON GRASS CHICKEN AND RICE ROLLS

4 lemon grass stems, white part only,
  halved lengthways
3 boneless, skinless chicken breasts,
  halved lengthways
2 tsp sesame oil
2 red chillies, seeded and chopped
10½ oz Chinese broccoli (gai larn), halved

10½ oz plain rice noodle rolls
  (see Hint)
reduced-sodium soy sauce, to serve
lime wedges, to serve

PREP TIME: 15 MINUTES
COOKING TIME: 10 MINUTES
SERVINGS: 4

Arrange the lemon grass in a steamer. Put the chicken on top, brush with the sesame oil and sprinkle with chilli. Cover with a lid. Sit the steamer over a wok or saucepan of boiling water and steam for 5 minutes, or until half cooked.

Put the Chinese broccoli and rice noodle rolls in another steamer of the same size and sit it on top of the steamer with the chicken. Cover with a lid and steam for a further 5 minutes, or until the chicken is cooked and the broccoli is tender. Cut the chicken into thick slices and serve with the broccoli, noodle rolls, small bowls of soy sauce and wedges of lime.

HINT:
• Rice noodle rolls are fresh blocks of thin rice noodles that have been rolled into a sausage shape. They are available from Asian food stores. If you cannot get them you can use fresh rice noodles, which are lower GI.

PEPPERED LAMB AND ASPARAGUS STIR-FRY WITH NOODLES

MUNG BEAN VERMICELLI IS LOW-GI AND TOGETHER WITH THE BEEF AND VEGETABLES, IS A GOOD CHOICE FOR PEOPLE WATCHING THEIR WEIGHT.

10½ oz dried mung bean vermicelli

2 tsp green peppercorns, finely chopped

3 garlic cloves, finely chopped

2 tsp canola oil

1 lb lean lamb fillets

canola oil spray

1 onion, cut into small wedges

4 tbsp dry sherry

1 green pepper, cut into strips

7 oz broccoli florets

16 small asparagus spears, trimmed and cut into bite-sized pieces

2 tbsp oyster sauce

garlic chives, cut into short lengths, to garnish

PREP TIME: 35 MINUTES + 20 MINUTES MARINATING + 10 MINUTES SOAKING

COOKING TIME: 30 MINUTES

SERVINGS: 4

Put the noodles in a large bowl and cover with warm water. Soak for 10 minutes, or until they are translucent. Transfer to a saucepan of boiling water and cook for 15 minutes, or until tender. Rinse under cold water, then drain. Use scissors to cut into shorter lengths.

To make the marinade, put the green peppercorns, garlic and oil in a large non-metallic bowl. Add the lamb and toss well to coat. Cover with plastic wrap and marinate for 20 minutes.

Trim the lamb and cut into bite-sized pieces. Heat a wok over high heat until slightly smoking. Add the lamb in small batches and stir-fry briefly until browned and just cooked. Remove from the wok and keep warm. Reheat the wok between batches.

Reheat the wok, spray with oil and stir-fry the onion and 2 teaspoons of the sherry for 1 minute. Add the pepper and a pinch of salt. Cover, steam for 2 minutes, add the broccoli, asparagus and the remaining sherry and stir-fry for 1 minute. Cover and steam for 3 minutes, or until the vegetables are just tender. Return the lamb to the pan, add the oyster sauce and stir to combine with the vegetables. Add the noodles and stir through until warmed. Serve garnished with the garlic chives.

HINT:
• People with diabetes or who are relatively inactive can serve themselves less vermicelli for lower calories.

nutrition per serving: Energy 479 Cal; Fat 7 g; Saturated fat 1.9 g; Protein 25.4 g; Carbohydrate 70.2 g; Fiber 4.1 g; Cholesterol 65 mg; Sodium 582 mg

BEEF WITH OYSTER SAUCE

READY IN A FLASH—THIS DISH IS GREAT WHEN YOU WANT TO EAT
HEALTHY MEALS BUT HAVE LITTLE TIME FOR COOKING. THIS IS A
GOOD SOURCE OF PROTEIN.

1½ tsp cornstarch
½ cup reduced-salt beef stock
1½ tbsp oyster sauce
1 tsp finely crushed garlic
1 tsp sugar
2 tsp canola oil
½ to 1 lb lean rump steak, finely sliced
9 oz green beans, topped and tailed, cut
    into 2 in lengths
1 small red pepper, sliced

⅔ cup bean sprouts
boiled basmati rice, to serve

PREP TIME: 15 MINUTES
TOTAL COOKING TIME: 10 MINUTES
SERVINGS: 4

Dissolve the cornstarch in a little of the stock. Mix with the remaining stock, oyster sauce, garlic and sugar and set aside.

Heat the wok until very hot, add the oil and swirl it around to coat the side. Add the beef in batches and stir-fry over high heat for 2 minutes, or until it browns.

Add the beans and pepper and stir-fry another minute.

Add the cornstarch mixture to the wok and cook until the sauce boils and thickens. Stir in the bean sprouts and serve immediately with the rice.

nutrition per serving: Energy 404 Cal; Fat 7.1 g; Saturated fat 2.1 g; Protein 26.7 g; Carbohydrate 54.4 g; Fiber 3.1 g; Cholesterol 56 mg; Sodium 516 mg

JUNGLE PORK CURRY

CURRY PASTE
8–10 large dried red chillies
1 tbsp shrimp paste
1 tsp white pepper
1 lemon grass stem, white part only, sliced
5 red Asian shallots, sliced
5 garlic cloves, crushed
1 tbsp finely chopped galangal
2 tsp finely grated fresh ginger
2 small cilantro roots, chopped

2 tsp canola oil
1 garlic clove, finely chopped, extra
about 1 lb lean pork fillet, thinly sliced
2 cups reduced-salt chicken stock
1/2 tbsp reduced-sodium soy sauce
2 to 3 Thai eggplants, quartered

1 cup green beans, cut into 1¼ in lengths
¼ cup sliced bamboo shoots
4 kaffir lime leaves, torn
1 small handful Thai basil leaves, plus extra
  to serve
1 long red chilli, seeded and julienned
boiled basmati rice, to serve

PREP TIME: 30 MINUTES + 10 MINUTES
  SOAKING
TOTAL COOKING TIME: 20 MINUTES
SERVINGS: 4

To make the curry paste, soak the dried chillies in boiling water for 10 minutes. Drain and chop. Wrap the shrimp paste in foil and toast in a hot wok for 1 minute on each side. Remove from the foil and put the shrimp paste in a food processor or blender with the chopped chilli and remaining paste ingredients. Process until smooth. Add a little water if necessary to form a smooth paste.

Heat a wok over medium heat, add the oil and swirl to coat. Add the garlic and 4 tablespoons of the curry paste and cook, stirring, for 1–2 minutes, or until fragrant. Add the pork and stir-fry for 2–3 minutes, or until browned. Pour in the stock and soy sauce, stir to combine, then bring to a boil. Add the eggplant, beans, bamboo shoots and lime leaves, reduce the heat and simmer for 5–8 minutes, or until the vegetables are tender but not soft. Remove from the heat and stir in the basil leaves. Garnish with the chilli strips and extra basil leaves and serve with the rice.

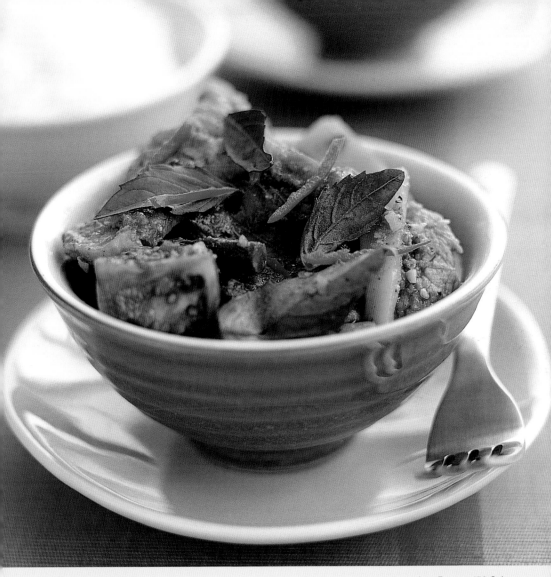

THIS AROMATIC THAI MEAL
PROVIDES PROTEIN, IRON AND
POTASSIUM. THE HOME-MADE
CURRY PASTE HAS LESS FAT
THAN COMMERCIAL VARIETIES.

nutrition per serving: Energy 453 Cal
Fat 6.5 g
Saturated fat 1.4 g
Protein 38.7 g
Carbohydrate 54.8 g
Fiber 5.5 g
Cholesterol 121 mg
Sodium 561 mg

BEEF IN BLACK BEAN SAUCE

THIS POPULAR CHINESE BEEF DISH SHOULD GIVE YOU AN ENERGY BOOST—
IT'S RICH IN IRON, ZINC AND CARBOHYDRATE.

2 garlic cloves, crushed
2 tsp grated fresh ginger
2 tbsp dry sherry
1 tbsp reduced-sodium soy sauce
1½ to 2 lbs lean beef rump steak
1 tsp cornstarch
2 tsp canola oil
2 onions, cut into wedges
1 large green pepper, cut
into strips

8½ oz canned sliced bamboo shoots,
drained and rinsed
2 tbsp canned black beans, rinsed and
chopped
boiled basmati rice, to serve

PREP TIME: 20 MINUTES + 1 HOUR
MARINATING
COOKING TIME: 30 MINUTES
SERVINGS: 4

To make the marinade, combine the garlic, ginger, sherry and soy sauce in a non-metallic bowl. Trim the meat, then slice across the grain into long, thin strips. Add to the marinade and toss to coat well. Cover with plastic wrap and refrigerate for at least 1 hour, turning occasionally. Drain the meat, reserving the marinade.

Meanwhile, to make the stir-fry sauce, mix the cornstarch and remaining marinade with 2 tablespoons water until smooth.

Heat a wok until very hot, add half the oil and swirl to coat. Add the meat in small batches and stir-fry briefly until browned but not cooked through. Remove from the wok and drain on paper towels. Reheat the wok between batches.

Heat the remaining oil in the wok and swirl to coat. Add the onion and pepper and stir-fry over high heat for 3 minutes, or until the onion is soft. Add the bamboo shoots and black beans, then cook for 1 minute.

Return the meat to the wok along with the stir-fry sauce and stir-fry over high heat until the meat is cooked through and the sauce has thickened. Serve immediately with the rice.

HINTS:
• Leftover black beans can be refrigerated for up to 2 weeks.
• For extra fiber and filling power, serve with brown rice instead of white rice.

nutrition per serving: Energy 542 Cal; Fat 11.6 g; Saturated fat 4.1 g; Protein 60.4 g; Carbohydrate 54.5 g; Fiber 3.5 g; Cholesterol 120 mg; Sodium 308 mg

MIDDLE-EASTERN CHICKEN WITH BULGUR

A NOURISHING MEAL THAT TASTES GREAT AND IS EASY TO MAKE, THIS DISH IS A GOOD WAY TO INCLUDE LOW-GI BULGUR AND CHICKPEAS IN YOUR DIET.

2 cups bulgur
2 skinless chicken breast fillets
2 tsp olive oil
1 red onion, thinly sliced
10½ oz canned chickpeas, drained and rinsed
½ cup unsalted pistachios
1 tomato, chopped

juice of 1 orange
4 tbsp finely chopped flat-leaf (Italian) parsley

PREP TIME: 15 MINUTES +
15 MINUTES SOAKING
COOKING TIME: 20 MINUTES
SERVINGS: 4

Put the bulgur in a bowl, cover with water and leave to soak for 15 minutes, or until the bulgur has softened. Drain and use clean hands to squeeze dry.

Meanwhile, trim the chicken and thinly slice. Heat a large frying pan over high heat, add half the oil and swirl to coat. Add the chicken in batches and stir-fry for 3–5 minutes, or until cooked. Remove from the pan and keep warm. Reheat the pan between batches.

Add the remaining oil to the pan and cook the onion, stirring, for 2 minutes, then add the chickpeas, pistachios and tomato. Cook, stirring, for 3–5 minutes, or until the chickpeas are warmed through.

Pour in the orange juice, return the chicken and its juices to the pan and cook until half the juice has evaporated. Stir in the parsley. Season with freshly ground black pepper and serve with the bulgur.

nutrition per serving: Energy 2457 kJ (589 Cal); Fat 13.7 g; Saturated fat 2.2 g; Protein 39.6 g; Carbohydrate 63.3 g; Fiber 20.7 g; Cholesterol 65 mg; Sodium 190 mg

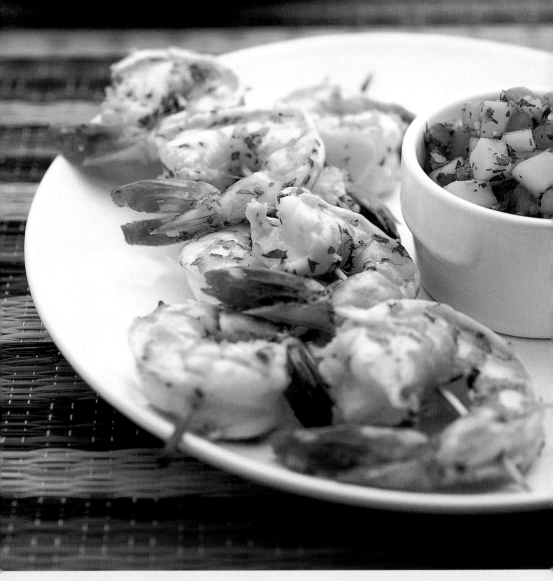

THIS COLORFUL DISH IS GREAT
IF YOU LOVE SEAFOOD. SHRIMP
PROVIDE PLENTY OF PROTEIN
WITH RELATIVELY FEW
CALORIES—BUT ENJOY IN
MODERATION AS THEY
CONTAIN CHOLESTEROL.

nutrition per serving: Energy 507 Cal
Fat 6.3 g
Saturated fat 0.9 g
Protein 38 g
Carbohydrate 69.3 g
Fiber 3.3 g
Cholesterol 226 mg
Sodium 547 mg

HONEY AND LIME SHRIMP KEBABS WITH MANGO SALSA

MANGO SALSA
2 tomatoes
1 small just-ripe mango, diced
½ small red onion, diced
1 small red chilli, seeded and finely
  chopped
grated zest and juice of 1 lime
2 tbsp chopped cilantro leaves

2 tbsp honey
1 small red chilli, seeded and finely
  chopped
1 tbsp olive oil

grated zest and juice of 2 limes
1 large garlic clove, crushed
¾ in piece fresh ginger, peeled and finely
  grated
1 tbsp chopped cilantro leaves
32 tiger or king shrimp, peeled and
  deveined, tails intact
boiled rice, to serve

PREP TIME: 25 MINUTES + 30 MINUTES
  SOAKING + 2 HOURS MARINATING
COOKING TIME: 5 MINUTES
SERVINGS: 4

Before you start cooking, soak eight bamboo skewers in cold water for 30 minutes. While the skewers are soaking, make the salsa. Score a cross in the base of each tomato and put them in a heatproof bowl. Cover with boiling water, leave for 30 seconds, then plunge in cold water and peel the skin away from the cross. Remove the seeds, dice the flesh, saving any juices, and put the tomato with all its juices in a bowl. Mix in the mango, onion, chilli, lime zest, lime juice and cilantro.

In a small bowl, whisk together the honey, chilli, oil, lime zest, lime juice, garlic, ginger and cilantro. Put the shrimp in a non-metallic dish, add the marinade and toss well. Cover and refrigerate for 2 or more hours, turning the shrimp occasionally.

Heat the grill or broiler to high. Thread 4 shrimp onto each skewer and grill for 4 minutes, or until pink and cooked through, turning halfway through cooking and basting regularly with the leftover marinade. Serve at once with the salsa and the rice.

HINT:
• When threading the shrimp on the skewers, don't squash them too closely together as they may not cook through properly.

FETTUCINE WITH SEARED TUNA AND ZUCCHINI

THIS LOW-FAT MEDITERRANEAN-STYLE DISH WITH A HINT OF ZESTY LEMON PROVIDES PLENTY OF PROTEIN, CARBOHYDRATE, NIACIN, POTASSIUM AND FOLATE, AND SOME IRON AND ZINC.

1 lb fettucine pasta
1 lb tuna steaks
olive oil spray
1 large red onion, cut into thin wedges
2 zucchini, sliced into 2¾ in long thin strips
1 garlic clove, chopped
6 small gherkins, rinsed and chopped

1 large handful flat-leaf (Italian) parsley,
  chopped
zest and juice of 1 large lemon
mixed-leaf salad, to serve (optional)

PREP TIME: 15 MINUTES
COOKING TIME: 20 MINUTES
SERVINGS: 4

Cook the pasta in a large saucepan of boiling water for 10 minutes, or until *al dente*. Drain, reserving 1 cup of the pasta water. Return the pasta to the saucepan.

Meanwhile, pat the fish dry with paper towels. Lightly spray a large, non-stick frying pan with the oil. Heat the oil, add the fish and cook for 2–3 minutes on each side, or until browned on the outside and still pink in the centre. Remove the fish from the pan. Set aside for a few minutes, then cut into ¾ in cubes.

Spray the frying pan with more oil and heat the pan. Add the onion, zucchini and garlic and cook for 2–3 minutes, or until softened. Stir in the gherkins, parsley, lemon zest and juice. Toss into the hot pasta together with the fish and enough of the reserved pasta water to moisten. Serve with a mixed-leaf salad.

nutrition per serving: Energy 609 Cal; Fat 9.5 g; Saturated fat 3.3 g; Protein 45.8 g; Carbohydrate 80.2 g; Fiber 5.2 g; Cholesterol 63 mg; Sodium 271 mg

PASTA WITH MEATBALLS

THIS DELICIOUS DISH IS RICH IN SLOW-RELEASE CARBOHYDRATE AND PROTEIN. LOW-GI, IT PROVIDES IRON AND ZINC, FOLATE AND POTASSIUM.

1 lb lean ground veal
1 onion, very finely chopped
4 garlic cloves, finely chopped
1 egg white, lightly beaten
1 cup fresh breadcrumbs
½ cup finely chopped parsley
¼ cup finely chopped oregano
olive oil spray
3 to 3½ lbs tomatoes, peeled, roughly chopped
2 onions, thinly sliced, extra

½ cup no-added-salt tomato paste
½ tsp sugar
12 oz penne
mixed-leaf salad, to serve (optional)

PREP TIME: 40 MINUTES
COOKING TIME: 1 HOUR 50 MINUTES
SERVINGS: 6

Combine the veal, onion, half the garlic, egg white, breadcrumbs, two-thirds of the parsley and 1 tablespoon of the oregano. Season well. Mix with your hands until well combined. Shape into small balls.

Heat a frying pan and spray with oil. Cook the meatballs in three batches over high heat for 4–5 minutes, or until browned, turning constantly. Remove from the pan.

Lightly spray the base of a large, deep non-stick saucepan with oil. Add the sliced onion and remaining garlic. Cook over low heat for 2–3 minutes, stirring. Add 2 tablespoons water, cover and cook for 5 minutes. Stir in the tomatoes and tomato paste. Simmer, covered, for 10 minutes, then uncover and simmer gently for 40 minutes. Add the meatballs, and simmer, covered, for 15–20 minutes, or until just cooked. Add the sugar, remaining parsley and oregano, and season with freshly ground black pepper.

Cook the pasta in a large saucepan of boiling water for 10 minutes, or until *al dente*, then drain. Serve with the hot meatballs and the salad.

nutrition per serving: Energy 454 Cal; Fat 8 g; Saturated fat 2.6 g; Protein 31.2 g; Carbohydrate 59.2 g; Fiber 7 g; Cholesterol 68 mg; Sodium 213 mg

PENNE WITH BACON, RICOTTA AND BASIL SAUCE

2 tsp olive oil

4 low-fat bacon slices (we used 97% fat-free), chopped

2–3 garlic cloves, crushed

1 onion, finely chopped

2 spring onions (scallions), finely chopped

1 cup low-fat ricotta cheese

3 handfuls basil, finely chopped, plus extra whole leaves, to garnish

12 oz penne

12 cherry tomatoes, halved

PREP TIME: 20 MINUTES

COOKING TIME: 15 MINUTES

SERVINGS: 4

Heat the oil in a frying pan, add the bacon, garlic, onion and spring onion and stir over medium heat for 5 minutes, or until cooked. Remove from the heat, stir in the ricotta and chopped basil and beat until smooth.

Cook the pasta in a large saucepan of boiling water for 10 minutes, or until *al dente*. Just prior to draining the pasta, add about 1 cup of the pasta cooking water to the ricotta mixture to thin the sauce. Add more water if you prefer an even thinner sauce. Season with freshly ground black pepper.

Drain the pasta and stir the ricotta sauce and tomato halves through the pasta. Garnish with extra basil and serve.

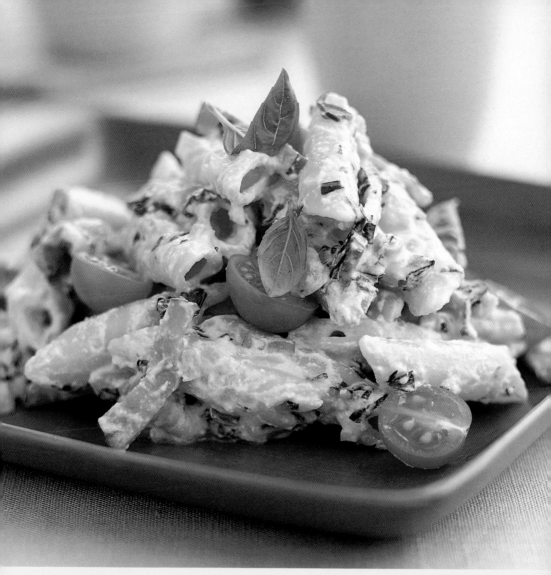

DELICIOUS FRESHLY PREPARED
BUT ALSO WHEN SERVED AS
LEFTOVERS, THIS ITALIAN
MEAL IS RICH IN FLAVOR
AND NUTRIENTS.

nutrition per serving: Energy 406 Cal
Fat 7.2 g
Saturated fat 2.1 g
Protein 21.3 g
Carbohydrate 61.7 g
Fiber 4.7 g
Cholesterol 8 mg
Sodium 516 mg

CHICKEN AND VEGETABLE LASAGNA

A REAL CROWD PLEASER, THIS VERSION OF LASAGNA IS MADE WITH CHICKEN AND LOTS OF VEGETABLES. IT'S LOW-GI AND CONTAINS MUCH LESS FAT THAN TRADITIONAL LASAGNA.

about 1 lb chicken breast fillets

olive oil spray

2 garlic cloves, crushed

1 onion, chopped

2 zucchini, chopped

2 celery stalks, chopped

2 carrots, chopped

1 medium peeled pumpkin or winter squash, diced

28 oz can reduced-salt diced tomatoes

2 sprigs thyme

2 bay leaves

2 tbsp no-added-salt tomato paste

½ cup dry white wine

2 tbsp chopped basil

1 lb spinach

1 lb low-fat cottage cheese

1 lb low-fat ricotta cheese

¼ cup skim milk

½ tsp ground nutmeg

⅓ cup grated parmesan cheese

12 lasagna sheets

PREP TIME: 45 MINUTES

TOTAL COOKING TIME: 1 HOUR 20 MINUTES

SERVINGS: 8

Preheat the oven to 350°F. Trim any excess fat from the chicken breasts, then finely mince in a food processor. Heat a large, deep, non-stick frying pan, spray lightly with oil and cook the chicken in batches until browned. Set aside. Add the garlic and onion to the pan and cook until softened. Return the chicken to the pan and add the zucchini, celery, carrot, pumpkin, tomato, thyme, bay leaves, tomato paste and wine. Simmer, covered, for 20 minutes. Remove the bay leaves and thyme, stir in the fresh basil and set aside.

Shred the spinach and set aside. Mix the cottage cheese, ricotta, skim milk, nutmeg and half the parmesan. Spoon a little of the tomato mixture over the base of a casserole dish and top with a single layer of pasta, top with half the remaining tomato mixture, then the spinach and spoon over half the cottage cheese mixture. Continue with another layer of pasta. Spread the remaining tomato mixture then the cottage cheese on top and sprinkle with parmesan. Bake for 40–50 minutes, or until golden. The top may puff up slightly but will settle on standing.

nutrition per serving: Energy 411 Cal; Fat 7.5 g; Saturated fat 3.2 g; Protein 40.4 g; Carbohydrate 39.7 g; Fiber 6.3 g; Cholesterol 53 mg; Sodium 299 mg

ITALIAN FISH ROLLS WITH SWEET POTATO

THIS FLAVORFUL MEAL IS A DELICIOUS WAY TO EAT FISH AND IS A GOOD SOURCE OF PROTEIN, IODINE, SELENIUM, BETA-CAROTENE AND B-GROUP VITAMINS. IT IS LOW-GI AND VERY LOW IN FAT.

1 large tomato

1 tbsp capers, drained and chopped

¼ cup stuffed green olives
   in brine, drained and chopped

3 tbsp finely chopped lemon thyme

¼ cup finely grated romano cheese

2 tsp finely grated lemon zest

¼ tsp freshly ground black pepper

8 thin white skinless fish fillets (about
   2 lbs) (see Hint)

1 cup dry white wine

2 tbsp lemon juice

3 tbsp lemon thyme, extra

2 bay leaves

2 large sweet potatoes, peeled
   and cut into 2 in pieces

PREP TIME: 30 MINUTES

COOKING TIME: 30 MINUTES

SERVINGS: 4–6

Preheat the oven to 315°F. Peel and chop the tomato and score a cross in the base. Cover with boiling water for 30 seconds, then plunge into cold water. Drain and peel away the skin from the cross. Cut in half and scoop out the seeds. Roughly chop the flesh and mix with the capers, olives, lemon thyme, cheese, lemon zest and freshly ground pepper in a small bowl.

Put the fillets, skinned side up, on a flat surface. Spread the tomato mixture evenly onto each fillet, then roll up tightly and secure with a toothpick or skewer. Place in a single layer in a shallow casserole dish.

Pour the combined wine, juice, lemon thyme and bay leaves over the fish, cover with foil and bake for 20 minutes, or until the fish is cooked and flakes easily when tested with a fork.

Meanwhile, cook the sweet potato in a large saucepan of boiling water for 10 minutes or until cooked. Drain and roughly mash. Season with freshly ground black pepper. Serve with the fish rolls.

HINT:
• Use bluegill, perch or snapper or ask your fishmonger for a suggestion.

nutrition per serve (6): Energy 281 Cal; Fat 5.1 g; Saturated fat 1.9 g; Protein 31.1 g; Carbohydrate 18.3 g; Fiber 3.9 g; Cholesterol 78 mg; Sodium 366 mg

113

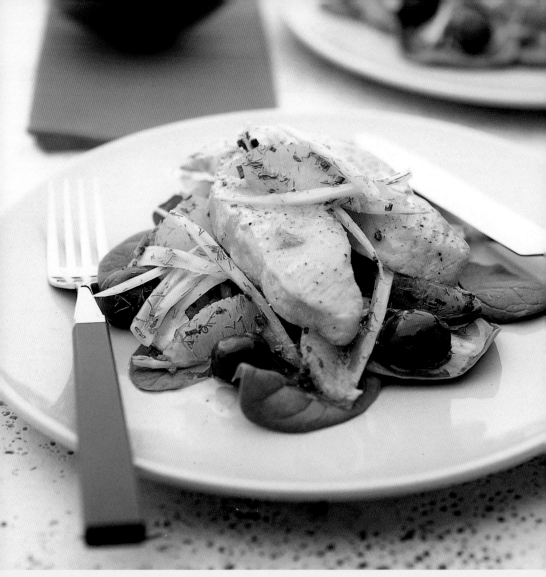

THIS TASTY DISH IS A GREAT
WAY TO INCLUDE THE
NUTRITIONAL BENEFITS OF
SALMON IN YOUR DIET. IT
CONTAINS OMEGA-3 FATTY
ACIDS, PROTEIN, POTASSIUM
AND PHOSPHORUS.

nutrition per serving: Energy 304 Cal
Fat 16.2 g
Saturated fat 3 g
Protein 26.9 g
Carbohydrate 10.4 g
Fiber 4.4 g
Cholesterol 65 mg
Sodium 171 mg

GRILLED SALMON WITH FENNEL AND ORANGE SALAD

FENNEL AND ORANGE SALAD
1 fennel bulb, with fronds
2 oranges, peeled and segmented
12 pitted black olives
1 tbsp snipped chives
1½ tbsp virgin olive oil
1 tbsp lemon juice
½ tsp dijon mustard
¼ tsp sugar

about 1 lb piece salmon fillet
olive oil spray
7 oz baby spinach leaves

PREP TIME: 20 MINUTES
COOKING TIME: 2 MINUTES
SERVINGS: 4

To prepare the salad, trim the fronds from the fennel bulb and finely chop up enough fronds to fill a tablespoon. Remove the stalks from the fennel and cut a ¼ in thick slice off the base of the bulb. Cut the bulb in half, then finely slice and toss in a large bowl with the chopped fronds, orange segments, olives and chives. In a separate bowl, whisk the oil with the lemon juice, mustard and sugar. Season to taste with freshly ground black pepper, pour over the fennel mixture and toss gently to coat.

Heat the grill or broiler to medium. Remove the bones and skin from the salmon and cut the flesh into ½ in thick slices. Lightly spray a grill tray with oil, put on the salmon slices, spray with more oil and season with freshly ground black pepper. Grill for 1–2 minutes, or until just cooked through.

Divide the spinach leaves among four large serving plates, top with the fennel and orange salad and arrange the salmon over the spinach. Serve warm.

HINT:
• Fennel bulbs are easily sliced using the slicing disc of a food processor.

LAMB CUTLETS WITH CANNELLINI BEAN PUREE

LEGUMES LIKE CANNELLINI BEANS ARE A GREAT FOOD TO INCLUDE IN A LOWER FAT DIET TO CONTROL YOUR BLOOD CHOLESTEROL BECAUSE THEY ARE LOW-GI, LOW IN FAT AND CHOLESTEROL FREE.

8 lean lamb cutlets

4 garlic cloves

1 tbsp chopped rosemary

2 tsp olive oil

28 oz canned cannellini beans, drained

1 tsp ground cumin

½ cup lemon juice

olive oil spray

2 tbsp balsamic vinegar

PREP TIME: 30 MINUTES + 1 HOUR
   REFRIGERATION

TOTAL COOKING TIME: 10 MINUTES

SERVINGS: 4

Trim the cutlets of excess fat from the outside edge and scrape the fat away from the bones. Put in a single layer in a shallow dish. Thinly slice 2 garlic cloves and mix with the rosemary, oil and some freshly ground black pepper. Pour over the meat, cover and refrigerate for 1 hour.

Rinse the beans and purée with the remaining garlic, the cumin and half the lemon juice in a food processor or blender. Transfer to a pan, then set aside.

Lightly spray a non-stick frying pan with oil and cook the cutlets over medium heat for 1–2 minutes on each side. Add the vinegar and cook for 1 minute, turning to coat. Remove the cutlets and cover to keep warm. Add the remaining lemon juice to the pan and simmer for 2–3 minutes, or until the sauce thickens slightly. Warm the purée over medium heat and serve with the cutlets.

nutrition per serving: Energy 312 Cal; Fat 11.6 g; Saturated fat 4.3 g; Protein 29.2 g; Carbohydrate 18.4 g; Fiber 9.3 g; Cholesterol 60 mg; Sodium 71 mg

STEAK SANDWICH WITH ONION RELISH

THIS IS ONE HEARTY (AND TASTY) SANDWICH THAT'S PACKED WITH LOTS OF NUTRIENTS, SUCH AS PROTEIN, NIACIN, PHOSPHORUS AND EASILY ABSORBED ZINC AND IRON.

RED ONION RELISH
1 tsp olive oil
2 red onions, thinly sliced
2 tbsp brown sugar
2 tbsp balsamic vinegar
1 tbsp chopped thyme

9 oz mixed mushrooms (flat, button, shiitake), sliced
olive oil spray

4 lean beef steaks, trimmed
3 large handfuls baby spinach leaves
ciabatta or sourdough bread
mixed-leaf salad, to serve (optional)

PREP TIME: 20 MINUTES
COOKING TIME: 25 MINUTES
SERVINGS: 4

To make the red onion relish, heat the oil in a saucepan. Add the onion and cook over low heat for 10 minutes, or until softened, taking care not to burn. Add the sugar and balsamic vinegar. Cook and stir often over low heat for 10–12 minutes, or until softened and slightly syrupy. Stir in the thyme.

Meanwhile, put the mushrooms and 1/2 cup water in a heavy-based frying pan. Bring to a boil, stirring to coat the mushrooms in the water. Simmer, covered, for 5 minutes, or until softened, making sure the mushrooms don't dry out. Stir once or twice. Remove the lid and increase the heat to allow the juice to evaporate. Season with freshly ground black pepper.

Lightly spray a chargrill pan or frying pan with the oil. Add the meat and cook for 1 minute on each side, or until cooked to your liking.

Very briefly microwave or steam the spinach until just wilted. Drain away any juices.

Slice the bread diagonally into 8 thick slices and toast. To serve, arrange 2 slices of bread on each plate. Top with the spinach, then the steak and mushrooms and finish with a dollop of the relish. Serve with a mixed-leaf salad to boost your intake of antioxidants.

nutrition per serving: Energy 435 Cal; Fat 9.8 g; Saturated fat 3.2 g; Protein 41.3 g; Carbohydrate 41.7 g; Fiber 6.2 g; Cholesterol 85 mg; Sodium 477 mg

SHISH KEBABS WITH ORZO SALAD

1 cup orzo
2 tsp extra virgin olive oil
2 tsp balsamic vinegar
½ tsp grated lemon zest
2 tsp lemon juice
2 handfuls arugula leaves
1½ tbsp shredded basil
½ small red onion, finely sliced

SHISH KEBABS
½ lb lean ground lamb
½ lb ground veal

1 onion, finely chopped
2 garlic cloves, crushed
1 tsp ground allspice
1 tsp ground cinnamon
olive oil spray

PREP TIME: 25 MINUTES + 30 MINUTES
REFRIGERATION TIME
COOKING TIME: 20 MINUTES
SERVINGS: 4

First, make the orzo salad. Bring a saucepan of water to a boil, add the orzo and cook for about 12 minutes, or until tender. Drain, rinse under cold water, then drain again. Put the orzo in a large bowl with the oil, vinegar, lemon zest, lemon juice, arugula, basil and onion. Mix well, season to taste with freshly ground black pepper and refrigerate until ready to serve.

To make the shish kebabs, put the lamb, veal, onion, garlic, allspice and cinnamon in a food processor or blender with a little pepper. Process until fine, but not mushy. Divide the mixture into eight equal portions, then roll into long sausage-shaped shish kebabs. Insert a long metal skewer through the middle of each shish kebab, pressing the mixture firmly onto the skewers. Refrigerate for 30 minutes to firm.

Preheat a barbecue grill plate, flat plate or chargrill pan to medium. Spray the hotplate with oil and grill the kebabs for about 8–10 minutes, or until cooked through, turning often. Serve warm with the orzo salad.

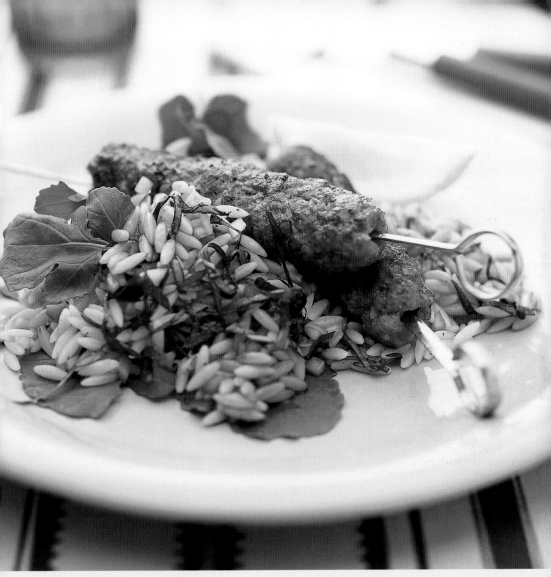

THESE MIDDLE-EASTERN
KEBABS ARE SURE TO BE A
FAVORITE WITH THE WHOLE
FAMILY. THEY ARE HIGH IN
PROTEIN, LOW-GI AND A GOOD
SOURCE OF IRON AND ZINC.

nutrition per serving: Energy 400 Cal
Fat 12.5 g
Saturated fat 4.2 g
Protein 32.9 g
Carbohydrate 36.9 g
Fiber 3 g
Cholesterol 94 mg
Sodium 111 mg

119

VEAL GOULASH

THIS TRADITIONAL HEARTY HUNGARIAN STEW IS A REAL CROWD PLEASER.
SLOW-COOKED WITH THE COMPLEX TASTE AND AROMA OF PAPRIKA, IT IS A
GREAT DISH TO COOK AND ENJOY ON A LAZY WEEKEND.

about 1 lb veal, cut into 1 in pieces
2 tbsp all-purpose flour
1 tbsp olive oil

olive oil spray
2 onions thinly sliced
2 garlic cloves, chopped
1 tbsp sweet Hungarian paprika
1 tsp ground cumin
15 oz canned reduced-salt diced tomatoes
2 carrots, sliced
1/2 red pepper, chopped
1/2 green pepper, chopped

1 cup reduced-salt beef stock
1/2 cup red wine
1/2 cup extra-light sour cream
chopped parsley, to garnish

PREP TIME: 25 MINUTES
TOTAL COOKING: TIME 2 HOURS
SERVINGS: 4

Put the veal and flour in a plastic bag and shake to coat the veal. Shake off any excess flour. Heat the oil in a large deep heavy-based pan over medium heat. Brown the meat well in batches, then remove the meat and set aside.

Reheat the pan and spray with olive oil. Cook the onion, garlic, paprika and cumin for 5 minutes, stirring frequently. Return the meat and any juices to the pan with the tomato, carrot and pepper. Cook and cover for 10 minutes.

Add the stock and wine and season with freshly ground black pepper. Stir well, then cover and simmer over very low heat for 1 1/2 hours. Stir in half the sour cream, season with more pepper if needed and serve garnished with parsley and the remaining sour cream.

HINT:
• This dish is delicious served with boiled new potatoes or noodles.

nutrition per serving: Energy 340 Cal; Fat 12.5 g; Saturated fat 4.2 g; Protein 33.3 g; Carbohydrate 16.1 g; Fiber 4.3 g; Cholesterol 103 mg; Sodium 424 mg

GIANT SALMON BALLS

YOU'LL BE BOWLED OVER BY THESE TASTY SALMON BALLS BECAUSE THEY
ARE OVEN-BAKED AND NOT DEEP-FRIED. TEAM THEM WITH A SALAD AND MAKE
A MEAL OF THEM.

3 potatoes, cut into 2 in cubes
$\frac{1}{2}$ cup long-grain rice
$\frac{1}{2}$ cup rolled oats
15 oz canned red salmon in spring water,
   drained and flaked
1 egg, lightly beaten
3 spring onions (scallions), chopped
2 tbsp lemon juice
2 tbsp sweet chilli sauce
1 cup fresh breadcrumbs

2 eggs, lightly beaten, extra
2 cups dry breadcrumbs
olive oil spray
lemon wedges, to serve
mixed-leaf salad, to serve

PREP TIME: 35 MINUTES + 30 MINUTES
   REFRIGERATION
COOKING TIME: 40 MINUTES
MAKES 8 BALLS

Boil, steam or microwave the potatoes until tender. Drain, mash and set aside to cool.
Cook the rice in a saucepan of boiling water for 10 minutes, or until tender. Drain and cool.

Put the potato, rice, oats, salmon, egg, spring onions, lemon juice, chilli sauce and fresh
breadcrumbs in a bowl, and mix together well. Season with freshly ground black pepper.

Divide the mixture into 8 portions and shape into balls. Dip in the egg, then in the dry
breadcrumbs. Place on a baking tray lined with baking paper, cover and refrigerate for
30 minutes.

Preheat the oven to 400°F. Spray the salmon balls lightly with the oil and bake for 30
minutes, or until crisp, golden and heated through. Serve with lemon wedges and a large
mixed-leaf salad.

nutrition per serving: Energy 343 Cal; Fat 9 g; Saturated fat 2.3 g; Protein 18 g; Carbohydrate 45.3 g;
Fiber 3.2 g; Cholesterol 96 mg; Sodium 348 mg

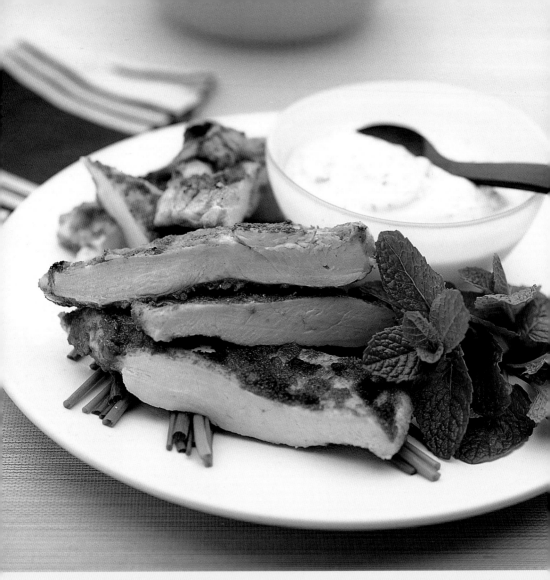

THESE CHICKEN SCHNITZELS
HAVE A TOUCH OF THE EXOTIC
ABOUT THEM, COATED IN
HERBS AND SPICES RATHER
THAN BREADCRUMBS.

nutrition per serving: Energy 516 Cal
Fat 8.9 g
Saturated fat 2.1 g
Protein 56.9 g
Carbohydrate 48.8 g
Fiber 3.7 g
Cholesterol 133 mg
Sodium 283 mg

SPICY CHICKEN SCHNITZELS

4 x 7 oz chicken breast fillets
½ tbsp ground coriander
½ tbsp ground cumin
¼ tsp chilli powder, or to taste
1 garlic clove, crushed
1 tbsp lemon juice
1 tbsp olive oil
1 cup low-fat plain yogurt
½ tsp harissa paste, or to taste
½ tsp sugar
2 tbsp finely chopped mint leaves, plus
extra sprigs, to serve

COUSCOUS SALAD
1 cup couscous
10 oz canned chickpeas, rinsed and drained
12 cherry tomatoes, halved
½ small red onion, thinly sliced

PREP TIME: 25 MINUTES + 15 MINUTES
STANDING
COOKING TIME: 10 MINUTES
SERVINGS: 4

Put the chicken breasts between two sheets of plastic wrap and flatten them with a mallet or rolling pin until ⅝ in thick.

In a small bowl, mix the ground coriander, cumin, chilli powder, garlic, lemon juice and oil together to form a paste. Thoroughly rub the paste all over the chicken fillets, then cover and leave to stand for 10 minutes.

To make the couscous salad, pour 1 cup boiling water over the in couscous in a bowl. Cover with plastic wrap and leave for 5 minutes then fluff up with a fork. Stir through chick peas, tomatoes and onion slices.

Heat the grill or broiler to high. Put the chicken on a lightly oiled grill tray and grill for 6–8 minutes, or until cooked through, turning once.

Meanwhile, blend 1 tablespoon of the yogurt in a bowl with the harissa and sugar. Stir in the remaining yogurt and mint, season to taste with freshly ground black pepper.

Garnish the chicken with the extra mint sprigs and serve with the yogurt mix and couscous.

HINT:
• These schnitzels are also delicious served cold or eaten in a wholegrain bread roll as a burger.

STUFFED BEEF FILLET

THIS NOURISHING DISH SHOWS HOW EASY IT IS TO EAT A VARIETY OF VEGETABLES IN ONE MEAL. IT'S A GOOD SOURCE OF PROTEIN, B GROUP VITAMINS, IRON AND ZINC.

1 tsp olive oil

2 French shallots, finely chopped

2¼ oz mushrooms, finely chopped

½ cup fresh whole-wheat breadcrumbs

1 tbsp thyme

1 tbsp wholegrain mustard

olive oil spray

1½ lbs lean beef fillet

8 to 10 new potatoes, cut into bite-sized chunks

4 corn cobs, each cut in 4 pieces

SAUCE

1 tsp orange zest

¾ cup orange juice

1 tbsp orange marmalade

1 tbsp wholegrain mustard

PREP TIME: 30 MINUTES

COOKING TIME: 55 MINUTES

SERVINGS: 4

Preheat the oven to 375°F. Heat the oil in a non-stick frying pan. Cook the shallots and mushrooms for 2 minutes, or until slightly softened. Put in a small bowl with the breadcrumbs and thyme leaves. Mix in the mustard and 2 teaspoons water to just moisten.

Cut along one side of the fillet to open out or create a butterfly. Spread the mushroom mixture over the surface. Enclose the filling and tie, at intervals, with string. Pat the meat dry with paper towels. Spray a heavy-based frying pan with oil. Heat and add the beef and cook on high heat until browned all over. Put in a roasting pan. Roast for 25 minutes, or until cooked to your liking. Remove the meat from the oven, cover with foil and rest. Remove the string.

Meanwhile, line a baking tray with baking paper. Put the potatoes in a large saucepan of boiling water. Cook for 5 minutes, or until partially cooked. Drain well. Put the potatoes on the prepared tray. Season with freshly ground black pepper and spray with oil. Bake for 15–20 minutes, or until crisp and cooked through. Cook the corn cobs in a saucepan of boiling water for 8 minutes, or until tender. Drain.

Add the sauce ingredients to the roasting pan. Stir to dissolve the marmalade and allow it to reduce a little. To serve, thickly slice the meat. Arrange the meat on plates, drizzle over a little of the sauce and serve with the potatoes and corn.

nutrition per serving: Energy 491 Cal; Fat 10.9 g; Saturated fat 3.6 g; Protein 40.3 g; Carbohydrate 52.8 g; Fiber 7.8 g; Cholesterol 100 mg; Sodium 199 mg

REDUCED-FAT MOUSSAKA

THIS REDUCED-FAT VERSION OF A GREEK FAVORITE MAKES A NOURISHING, LOW-GI MEAL.

2 to 3 eggplants
olive oil spray
2 onions, finely chopped
3 large garlic cloves, crushed
½ tsp ground allspice
1 tsp ground cinnamon
about 1 lb lean ground lamb
2 tbsp no-added-salt tomato paste
½ cup red wine
28 oz canned reduced-salt tomatoes
3 tbsp chopped parsley
4 oz low-fat cheddar cheese

1½ tbsp olive or canola oil margarine
⅓ cup flour
1½ cups skim milk
⅔ cup low-fat ricotta
pinch ground nutmeg

PREP TIME: 30 MINUTES
COOKING TIME: 1½ HOURS
SERVINGS: 6

Preheat the oven to 350°F. Cut the eggplant into ¼ in thick slices. Spray the eggplant with the oil and grill or broil under a preheated grill or broiler for 4 minutes on each side, or until golden.

Heat a large, non-stick saucepan and lightly spray with oil. Cook the onions for 3–4 minutes, or until softened. Add the garlic, allspice and cinnamon and cook for 1 minute. Add the lamb and cook for 3–4 minutes, or until cooked. Add the tomato paste, wine and tomatoes. Bring to a boil, then reduce the heat and simmer for 30–35 minutes, stirring occasionally, or until most of the liquid has evaporated. Stir in the parsley and season with freshly ground black pepper.

To make the white sauce, grate the cheese. Melt the margarine in a saucepan over medium heat. Stir in the flour and cook for 1 minute. Remove from the heat and gradually stir in the milk. Return to the heat and stir constantly until the sauce boils and thickens. Reduce the heat and simmer for 2 minutes. Stir through the ricotta and nutmeg until smooth and season with pepper.

Spoon half the meat sauce over the base of a 9 x 13 in ovenproof dish. Cover with half of the eggplant. Spoon over the remaining meat sauce and cover with the remaining eggplant. Spread over the sauce and sprinkle with the cheese. Bake for 30 minutes, or until golden. Stand for 5 minutes before serving.

nutrition per serving: Energy 347 Cal; Fat 12.2 g; Saturated fat 4.4 g; Protein 31.4 g; Carbohydrate 20.8 g; Fiber 7.1 g; Cholesterol 65 mg; Sodium 282 mg

POACHED SALMON KEDGEREE

2 eggs

3 cups reduced-salt fish or chicken stock

1/2 cup dry white wine

1/2 lemon, sliced

7 oz salmon fillets

1 tsp canola oil margarine

1 large red onion, chopped

2 tbsp mild curry powder

2 tsp ground turmeric

1 1/2 cups basmati rice

1/2 cup golden raisins

1 large handful flat-leaf (Italian) parsley,
   finely chopped

1 lemon, cut into 4 wedges, to serve
   (optional)

fruit chutney, to serve (optional)

mixed-leaf salad, to serve (optional)

PREP TIME: 20 MINUTES

COOKING TIME: 40 MINUTES

SERVINGS: 4

Put the eggs in a saucepan, cover with water and bring to a boil. Boil for 5 minutes, drain and cool quickly in cold water. Peel and chop roughly.

Heat a heavy-based frying pan that is 3 in deep and 10 in in diameter across the base. Add the stock, wine and lemon slices and heat, then add the fish. Lower the heat and simmer for 8 minutes, or until just cooked through. Place the fish on a plate, remove the skin and roughly flake with a fork. Strain the stock into a jug to measure 3 cups. Set aside. Wipe out the pan.

Heat the butter in the frying pan, add the onion and cook for 2 minutes, or until softened. Add the curry powder, the turmeric and rice. Stir to combine and cook for 1 minute.

Stir in the reserved stock. Bring to a boil, lower the heat, cover and simmer for 20 minutes, or until the rice is cooked and the liquid has been absorbed.

Gently stir the chopped egg, fish, raisins and half of the parsley through the rice. Top with the remaining parsley and lemon wedges on the side, if using. Serve with a little fruit chutney and a mixed-leaf salad.

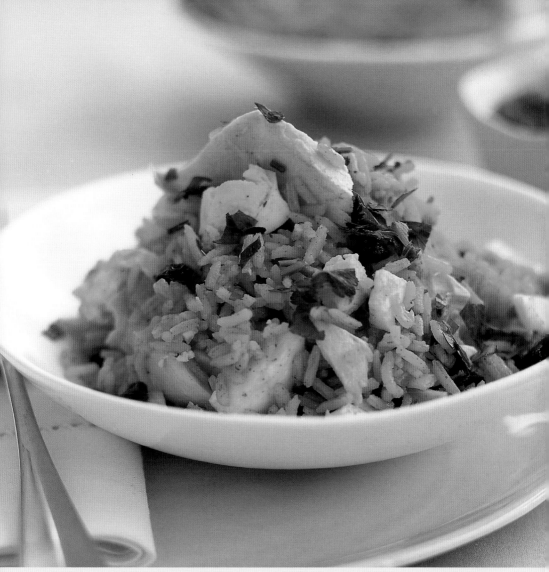

A SPICED DISH COMBINING
GOOD-QUALITY PROTEIN FROM
EGGS AND SALMON WITH LOW-GI
CARBOHYDRATE FROM BASMATI RICE.
THIS MEAL ALSO PROVIDES SOME
IRON, ESSENTIAL OMEGA-3 FATTY
ACIDS, NIACIN AND POTASSIUM.

nutrition per serving: Energy 569 Cal
Fat 11.3 g
Saturated fat 2.7 g
Protein 32.2 g
Carbohydrate 77.2 g
Fiber 3.4 g
Cholesterol 149 mg
Sodium 572 mg

SHEPHERD'S PIE

A REDUCED-FAT VERSION OF AN OLD FAVORITE, THIS HEARTY PIE IS JUST AS DELICIOUS AS THE REGULAR VERSION.

2 to 3 potatoes
6 large garlic cloves, peeled
4 tbsp skim milk
olive oil spray
1 large onion, finely chopped
3 large garlic cloves, crushed
2 celery sticks, finely chopped
2 carrots, diced
1 to 2 lbs lean ground lamb
1½ tbsp all-purpose flour
2 tbsp no-added-salt tomato paste
2 tsp chopped thyme
2 tsp chopped rosemary

2 bay leaves
1¼ cups reduced-salt beef stock
1 tbsp worcestershire sauce
pinch ground nutmeg
mixed-leaf salad, to serve (optional)

PREP TIME: 20 MINUTES
COOKING TIME: 45 MINUTES
SERVINGS: 6

Preheat the oven to 350°F. Cut the potatoes into chunks and cook in a large saucepan of boiling water with the whole garlic cloves for 10–15 minutes, or until tender. Drain well and return to the saucepan. Mash the potato and garlic with a potato masher until smooth. Stir through the milk and season with freshly ground black pepper.

Heat a frying pan over medium heat, then spray with oil. Add the onion, crushed garlic, celery and carrot and cook for 5 minutes, or until the vegetables begin to soften (add water if needed). Remove from the pan.

Add the lamb and cook over a high heat until well browned, breaking up any lumps with the back of a spoon. Add the flour and cook for 1–2 minutes. Return the vegetables to the pan with the tomato paste, herbs, bay leaf, stock, sauce and nutmeg and bring to a boil. Reduce the heat and simmer for 5 minutes, or until thickened.

Pour the lamb mixture into a 4 cup ovenproof dish. Spoon the potato over the top, smoothing the surface, then fluff with a fork. Bake for 25–30 minutes, or until lightly golden and crusty. Serve with a mixed-leaf salad.

nutrition per serving: Energy 357 Cal; Fat 9.8 g; Saturated fat 4.1 g; Protein 32.9 g; Carbohydrate 30.7 g; Fiber 5.6 g; Cholesterol 87 mg; Sodium 383 mg

MEATLOAF

PREPARING A FAMILY DINNER DOESN'T HAVE TO BE HARD WORK. MEATLOAF IS A GREAT WAY TO GET CHILDREN TO EAT VEGETABLES—SIMPLY GRATE THEM AND ADD THEM TO THE MIXTURE WHERE THEY WILL HARDLY BE NOTICED.

1 small sweet potato

1 carrot

canola or olive oil spray

2 onions, finely chopped

2 garlic cloves, crushed

1½ cups fresh wholegrain breadcrumbs

2 tbsp chopped parsley

about 1 lb lean ground beef

2 tbsp worcestershire sauce

1 tsp dried basil

1 tbsp no-added-salt tomato paste

10½ oz canned chickpeas, drained
    and rinsed

1 egg, lightly beaten

1 cup button mushrooms, thinly sliced

14 oz canned reduced-salt tomatoes

1 tbsp dry white wine

1 tsp brown sugar

mixed leaf salad, to serve

PREP TIME: 20 MINUTES

COOKING TIME: 1 HOUR 20 MINUTES

SERVINGS: 6

Preheat the oven to 400°F. Coarsely grate the sweet potato and carrot.

Heat a non-stick frying pan over medium heat, then spray with the oil. Add the onion and cook, stirring, for 2 minutes. Add 1 tablespoon water to prevent sticking, then add the garlic and stir for 3 minutes, or until the onion is golden brown. Set aside to cool completely.

Use your hands to thoroughly mix together the breadcrumbs, parsley, beef, Worcestershire sauce, basil, tomato paste, grated sweet potato and carrot and the cooled onion mixture. Mix in the chickpeas, egg and mushrooms. Season with freshly ground black pepper. Transfer to a 4½ x 8 in non-stick loaf pan (or loaf pan lined with baking paper, pressing gently into the tin and smoothing the top.

To make the tomato sauce, push the undrained tomatoes through a sieve, then discard the contents of the sieve. Add the wine and sugar to the tomato mixture, then stir well. Spoon 3 tablespoons of the sauce over the meatloaf and bake for 15 minutes. Spoon another 3 tablespoons of sauce over the meatloaf, reduce the oven temperature to 375°F and bake for 1 hour 10 minutes, basting occasionally with sauce. Slice and serve with any remaining sauce and a mixed-leaf salad.

nutrition per serving: Energy 271 Cal; Fat 8.5 g; Saturated fat 2.9 g; Protein 23.9 g; Carbohydrate 21.6 g; Fiber 5 g; Cholesterol 74 mg; Sodium 355 mg

VEGETARIAN MEALS

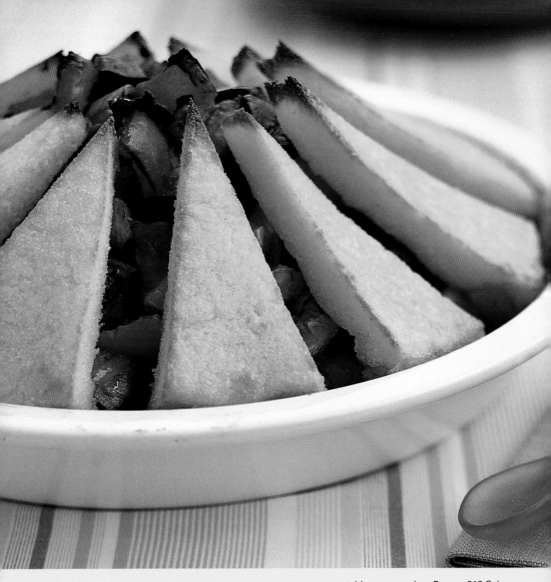

THIS COLORFUL DISH MAKES A
GREAT VEGETARIAN STARTER OR
CELEBRATORY MEAL. IF PREPARING
AS A MAIN MEAL, SERVE WITH A
DOLLOP OF YOGURT OR SOME
CHEESE FOR EXTRA CALCIUM
AND PROTEIN.

nutrition per serving: Energy 218 Cal
Fat 7.4 g
Saturated fat 2.3 g
Protein 8.9 g
Carbohydrate 26 g
Fiber 5.4 g
Cholesterol 8 mg
Sodium 366 mg

VEGETABLE AND POLENTA PIE

1⅓ cups reduced-salt vegetable stock

1 cup coarse polenta

½ cup finely grated parmesan cheese

1 tbsp olive oil

1 large onion, chopped

2 garlic cloves, crushed

2 eggplants

1 large red pepper, diced

2 zucchini, thickly sliced

5½ oz button mushrooms, cut
   into quarters

14 oz canned reduced-salt diced tomatoes

3 tsp balsamic vinegar

olive oil, for brushing

PREP TIME: 25 MINUTES + REFRIGERATION

COOKING TIME: 50 MINUTES

SERVINGS: 6

Line a 9 in round cake pan with foil. Pour the stock and 1½ cups water into a saucepan and bring to a boil. Add the polenta in a thin stream and stir over low heat for 5 minutes, or until the liquid is absorbed and the mixture is thick and comes away from the side of the pan. Remove the pan from the heat and stir in the cheese until it melts all through the polenta. Spread into the pan, smoothing the surface as much as possible. Refrigerate until set.

Preheat the oven to 400°F. Heat the oil in a large saucepan and add the onion. Cook over medium heat, stirring occasionally, for 3 minutes, or until soft. Add the garlic and cook for 1 minute. Add the eggplant, pepper, zucchini, mushrooms and tomatoes. Bring to a boil, then reduce the heat and simmer, covered, for 20 minutes, or until the vegetables are tender. Stir occasionally. Stir in the vinegar, then season with freshly ground black pepper.

Transfer the vegetable mixture to a 9 in pie dish, piling it up slightly in the center.

When the polenta has set, turn it out of the pan, peel off the foil and cut into 12 wedges. Arrange, smooth side down, in a single layer, over the vegetables—don't worry about any gaps. Brush lightly with olive oil and bake for 20 minutes, or until lightly brown and crisp.

MIDDLE-EASTERN POTATO CASSEROLE

THIS DELICIOUS DISH IS EASY TO PUT TOGETHER AND EVEN EASIER TO EAT. IT'S A LOVELY MEAL TO SHARE WITH FRIENDS.

¼ tsp saffron threads

3 to 4 medium potatoes (about 2 lbs), cut into large cubes

1 tsp olive oil

1 small onion, sliced

½ tsp ground turmeric

½ tsp ground coriander

1 cup reduced-salt vegetable stock

1 garlic clove, crushed

¼ cup raisins

1 tsp chopped flat-leaf (Italian) parsley

1 tsp chopped cilantro leaves

PREP TIME: 10 MINUTES

TOTAL COOKING TIME: 35 MINUTES

SERVINGS: 4

Soak the saffron in 1 tablespoon of hot water. Put the potatoes in a saucepan of cold, salted water. Bring to a boil and cook until tender but still firm. Drain and set aside.

Heat the oil in a separate saucepan, add the onion, turmeric and ground coriander and cook over low heat for 5 minutes, or until the onion is soft.

Add the potato, vegetable stock and garlic. Bring to a boil, then reduce the heat and simmer for 10 minutes.

Add the saffron with its soaking water and the raisins, and cook for 10 minutes, or until the potato is soft and the sauce has reduced and thickened. Stir in the parsley and cilantro.

HINT:
• This dish is delicious served with couscous.

nutrition per serving: Energy 219 Cal; Fat 1.8 g; Saturated fat 0.3 g; Protein 6.7 g; Carbohydrate 40.8 g; Fiber 5.1 g; Cholesterol 0 mg; Sodium 271 mg

MOROCCAN VEGETABLE TAGINE WITH COUSCOUS

THIS EXOTIC MIDDLE-EASTERN DISH PROVIDES A SATISFYING ALTERNATIVE TO RICE AND PASTA DISHES.

2 tsp oil
2 onions, chopped
1 tsp ground ginger
2 tsp ground paprika
2 tsp ground cumin
1 cinnamon stick
pinch of saffron threads
about 3 lbs mixed vegetables, peeled, and
cut into large chunks (carrot, eggplant,
sweet potato, parsnip, potato, pumpkin
or winter squash)
½ preserved lemon, rinsed, pith and flesh
removed, thinly sliced
15 oz canned reduced-salt peeled
tomatoes
1 cup reduced-salt vegetable stock

3 ½ oz dried pears, halved
2 ¼ oz pitted prunes
2 zucchini, cut into large chunks
10 oz instant couscous
1 tbsp olive oil
3 tbsp chopped flat-leaf (Italian) parsley
⅓ cup almonds

PREP TIME: 25 MINUTES
TOTAL COOKING TIME: 1 HOUR
SERVINGS: 4–6

Preheat the oven to 350°F. Heat the oil in a large saucepan or ovenproof dish, add the onion and cook over medium heat for 5 minutes, or until soft. Add the spices and cook for 3 minutes.

Add the vegetables and cook, stirring, until coated with the spices and the outsides begin to soften. Add the lemon, tomatoes, stock, pears and prunes. Cover, transfer to the oven and cook for 30 minutes. Add the zucchini and cook for 15–20 minutes, or until the vegetables are tender.

Cover the couscous with the olive oil and 2 cups boiling water, cover and leave until all the water has been absorbed. Fluff with a fork.

Remove the cinnamon stick from the vegetables, then stir in the parsley. Serve on a large platter with the couscous formed in a ring and the vegetable tagine in the center, sprinkle with almonds.

nutrition per serving (6): Energy 461 Cal; Fat 7.7 g; Saturated fat 0.8 g; Protein 14.3 g; Carbohydrate 78.4 g; Fiber 10.6 g; Cholesterol 0 mg; Sodium 283 mg

HARISSA WITH VEGETABLE COUSCOUS

HARISSA
3 dried bird's eye chilies
3 large garlic cloves
1 tsp coriander seeds
½ tsp ground cumin
¼ cup reduced-salt puréed tomatoes
1 tbsp extra virgin olive oil
1 tbsp no-added-salt tomato paste

2 tbsp roughly chopped cilantro leaves
2 tbsp roughly chopped mint
1 cup Greek-style low-fat yogurt
1⅔ cups couscous
2 tsp olive oil
1 large onion, halved and thinly sliced
3 zucchini, thinly sliced

2 large carrots, cut into fine matchsticks
   ¾ in long
14 oz canned chickpeas, rinsed
   and drained
⅓ cup golden raisins
¼ cup toasted slivered almonds
2 tbsp baby capers, rinsed and
   squeezed dry

PREP TIME: 20 MINUTES
COOKING TIME: 10 MINUTES
SERVINGS: 4–6

To make the harissa, put the chilies, garlic, coriander seeds and cumin in a mini processor or blender. Blend for 30 seconds, or until roughly ground. Add the pureed tomato, olive oil and tomato paste and blend for 12–15 seconds, or until smooth.

Put the cilantro, mint and yogurt in a small bowl and mix to combine.

Prepare the couscous according to the manufacturer's instructions. Cover and set aside. Heat the oil in a large frying pan over medium heat. Add the onion and fry for 5–6 minutes, or until softened. Add the zucchini and carrot and fry for 5 minutes, or until just tender and beginning to brown. Stir in the chickpeas and raisins. Add the couscous, stirring gently until well combined.

Divide the couscous mixture among serving plates and sprinkle with the toasted almonds and capers. Serve accompanied by the harissa and herbed yogurt, to be added as desired.

HINT:
• Store the harissa, covered with a thin layer of olive oil in an airtight container, in the refrigerator for 7–10 days.

136

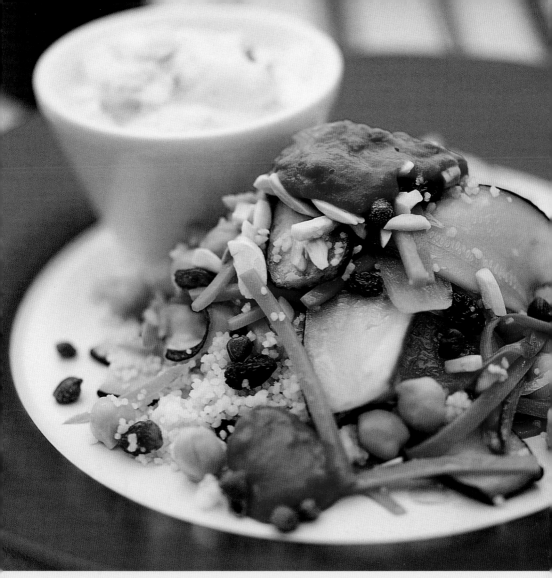

THIS COLORFUL DISH IS
A GREAT WAY TO INCLUDE
LEGUMES IN YOUR DIET, WHICH
CONTAIN PROTEIN, CALCIUM
AND GOOD AMOUNTS OF IRON.

nutrition per serving: Energy 380 Cal
Fat 8.7 g
Saturated fat 1.1 g
Protein 14.5 g
Carbohydrate 57.4 g
Fiber 6.2 g
Cholesterol 2 mg
Sodium 195 mg

137

CHICKPEA CURRY

THIS MILD BUT FLAVORFUL CURRY IS SURE TO SATISFY, BUT YOU NEED TO PLAN IN ADVANCE SO THAT THE CHICKPEAS CAN SOAK OVERNIGHT.

1 cup dried chickpeas

2 tsp oil

2 onions, finely chopped

2 large tomatoes, chopped

½ tsp ground coriander

1 tsp ground cumin

1 tsp chili powder

¼ tsp ground turmeric

1 tsp channa masala (see Hint)

1 small white onion, sliced, extra, to serve

mint and cilantro leaves, to garnish

boiled rice, to serve (optional)

PREP TIME: 15 MINUTES + OVERNIGHT
    SOAKING

TOTAL COOKING TIME: 1 HOUR 15 MINUTES

SERVINGS: 6

Put the chickpeas in a bowl, cover with water and leave to soak overnight. Drain, rinse, and put in a large saucepan. Cover with plenty of water and bring to a boil, then reduce the heat and simmer for 40 minutes, or until soft. Drain.

Heat the oil in a large saucepan, add the onion and cook over medium heat for 15 minutes, or until golden brown. Add the tomato, ground coriander and cumin, chili powder, turmeric and channa masala, and 2 cups water and cook for 10 minutes, or until the tomato is soft. Add the chickpeas, season with freshly ground pepper and cook for 7–10 minutes, or until the sauce thickens. Garnish with sliced onion and fresh mint and cilantro leaves, and serve with rice.

HINT:
• Channa (chole) masala is a spice blend available at Indian food stores. Garam masala can be used as a substitute but the flavor will be a little different.

nutrition per serving: Energy 176 Cal; Fat 4 g; Saturated fat 0.5 g; Protein 8.5 g; Carbohydrate 20 g; Fiber 8.1 g; Cholesterol 0 mg; Sodium 22 mg

WILD RICE WITH PUMPKIN

THIS TASTY DISH IS RELATIVELY EASY TO COOK. WILD RICE IS MUCH HIGHER IN PROTEIN THAN REGULAR RICE AND IS ALSO A GOOD SOURCE OF NIACIN.

1 cup wild rice, rinsed

10½ oz Japanese or sugar pumpkin, skin on, cut into ½ x 2½ in wedges

14 oz canned chickpeas, drained and rinsed

8 spring onions (scallions), finely sliced

⅓ cup currants

½ cup pistachio nuts, roughly chopped

1 tsp garam masala

3 tbsp pumpkin seeds

1 tbsp olive oil

2 tsp finely grated orange zest

1 large handful cilantro leaves

1 large handful mint, torn

PREP TIME: 20 MINUTES

COOKING TIME: 40 MINUTES

SERVINGS: 4–6

Put the rice in a small saucepan over medium–high heat, add 2½ cups water and cover with a lid. Bring to a boil, then reduce the heat to low and simmer for 30–35 minutes, or until all of the liquid has been absorbed and the rice is cooked but still *al dente*.

Line a steamer with baking paper and punch with holes. Arrange the pumpkin on top and cover with a lid. Sit the steamer over a saucepan or wok of boiling water and steam for 5 minutes, or until the pumpkin is tender when pierced with a sharp knife. Set aside to cool a little.

Put the chickpeas, spring onion, currants, pistachios, garam masala, pumpkin seeds, oil, orange zest, cilantro and mint leaves in a large bowl and season with freshly ground black pepper. Add the steamed rice and pumpkin wedges and toss gently to combine. Arrange the salad in a bowl or on a platter and serve warm.

nutrition per serving (6): Energy 310 Cal; Fat 13 g; Saturated fat 1.8 g; Protein 11.2 g; Carbohydrate 34.2 g; Fiber 6.7 g; Cholesterol 0 mg; Sodium 113 mg

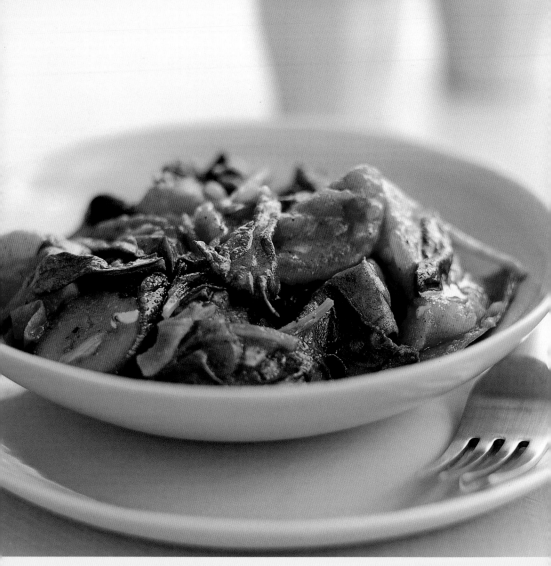

THIS SPICY DISH CONTAINS
EGGPLANT, WHICH IS A GREAT
VEGETABLE TO INCLUDE IN A
LOW-CHOLESTEROL DIET. IT
IS LOW IN FAT AND SODIUM
AND IS CHOLESTEROL FREE.

nutrition per serving: Energy 313 Cal
Fat 5.7 g
Saturated fat 0.7 g
Protein 7.6 g
Carbohydrate 53.2 g
Fiber 5.1 g
Cholesterol 0 mg
Sodium 24 mg

CURRIED EGGPLANT STIR-FRY

1 tbsp vegetable oil
½–1 long green chili, finely sliced
4 shallots, chopped
2 garlic cloves, finely sliced
2–3 tsp curry powder, to taste
2 slender eggplants, cut diagonally into
  ½ in slices
3 vine-ripened tomatoes, each cut into
  8 wedges

1½ cups baby spinach leaves
boiled basmati rice, to serve

PREP TIME: 15 MINUTES
COOKING TIME: 15 MINUTES
SERVINGS: 4

Heat the oil in a large wok and swirl to coat. Add the green chili, shallots and garlic and stir-fry over high heat for 1 minute. Stir in the curry powder and stir-fry for 1 minute.

Add the eggplant and stir-fry for 3 minutes, or until the eggplant has softened a little. Add the tomato and ½ cup water. Cover the wok and cook for 10 minutes, or until the eggplant is cooked, stirring occasionally. Stir in the spinach leaves and cook for 1 minute, or until wilted. Serve immediately with boiled rice.

CHILI TOFU STIR-FRY

TOFU IS A GREAT INGREDIENT TO CARRY FLAVORS, SOAKING UP THE COOKING JUICES IN A DISH. IT IS HIGH IN PROTEIN AND CONTAINS SOME IRON.

1 tbsp canola oil
1 tsp bottled crushed chili
2 tsp grated fresh ginger
2 garlic cloves, crushed
9 oz firm tofu, cut into cubes
8 spring onions (scallions), sliced on the diagonal
6 oz fresh baby corn, halved lengthways
1 handful snowpeas, topped and tailed
16 oz egg noodles
¼ cup cashew nuts
1 tbsp reduced-sodium soy sauce

½ cup reduced-salt vegetable stock
1 handful cilantro leaves

PREP TIME: 15 MINUTES
COOKING TIME: 15 MINUTES
SERVINGS: 4

Heat the oil in a wok over medium heat and swirl to coat. Add the chili, ginger and garlic and stir-fry for about 2–3 minutes, or until aromatic. Add the tofu cubes, spring onion and baby corn and stir-fry for 2–3 minutes.

Add the snowpeas, noodles and cashews and cook, stirring, for 3–5 minutes, or until the vegetables are almost tender. Stir in the soy sauce and stock, then bring to a boil and simmer for 2 minutes, or until slightly reduced. Stir in the cilantro and serve immediately.

nutrition per serving: Energy 381 Cal; Fat 15.5 g; Saturated fat 2.1 g; Protein 16.8 g; Carbohydrate 41.1 g; Fiber 7.3 g; Cholesterol 0 mg; Sodium 524 mg

PUMPKIN BHAJI

BHAJIS ARE POPULAR INDIAN VEGETABLE DISHES. THIS ONE IS MADE WITH PUMPKIN, WHICH CONTAINS VITAMIN A AND ANTIOXIDANT CAROTENOIDS, PARTICULARLY ALPHA- AND BETA-CAROTENES.

1 tbsp vegetable oil
1 tsp yellow mustard seeds
1 onion, finely chopped
1 tsp grated fresh ginger
1 green chili, seeded and chopped
1 tsp ground coriander
½ tsp garam masala
½ tsp ground turmeric
½ tsp ground cumin
½ tsp chili flakes

1 large pumpkin or winter squash, peeled, seeded and cut into 1¼ in cubes
15 oz canned reduced-salt diced tomatoes
1 tsp brown sugar
3 tbsp low-fat plain yogurt
cilantro leaves, to serve
boiled basmati rice, to serve

PREP TIME: 20 MINUTES
COOKING TIME: 35 MINUTES
SERVINGS: 4

Heat the oil in a large wok and cook the mustard seeds until they just start to pop. Add the onion, ginger and chili and stir-fry for 2 minutes. Add the coriander, garam masala, turmeric, cumin and chili flakes and stir-fry for 1 minute, or until aromatic.

Stir in the pumpkin, chopped tomatoes, sugar and ½ cup water. Bring to a boil, then reduce the heat and simmer, covered, for 30 minutes, or until the pumpkin is tender. Stir occasionally. Gently fold in the yogurt and scatter with cilantro leaves before serving with boiled rice.

nutrition per serving: Energy 384 Cal; Fat 6.5 g; Saturated fat 1.3 g; Protein 10.8 g; Carbohydrate 66 g; Fiber 5 g; Cholesterol 1 mg; Sodium 37 mg

ASIAN GREENS WITH CHILI AND COCONUT MARINADE

MARINADE
¼ cup shredded coconut
2 garlic cloves, roughly chopped
¾ in piece ginger, roughly chopped
1 shallot, roughly chopped
1 small red chili, sliced
2 tbsp canola oil
1 tbsp rice vinegar
2 tsp fish sauce
1 tsp brown sugar
2 spring onions (scallions), sliced

2 bunches Asian green vegetables
boiled rice, to serve (optional)

PREP TIME: 25 MINUTES + 1 HOUR
   MARINATING
COOKING TIME: 10 MINUTES
SERVINGS: 4

To make the marinade, heat a dry frying pan over medium heat. Add the shredded coconut and fry, stirring, for 3–4 minutes, or until brown. Transfer the coconut to a spice mill or mini processor, add the garlic, ginger, shallot and chili and blend until finely chopped. Add 1 tablespoon of oil, vinegar, fish sauce and sugar and blend in short bursts until blended. Transfer to a large bowl and stir in the spring onion.

Slice the Asian greens into 3¼ in lengths and divide these into stems and leaves. Heat a wok or large frying pan over medium–high heat and add the remaining oil. Add the vegetable stems and stir-fry for 1 minute. Add the vegetable leaves and stir-fry for 45–60 seconds, or until they wilt and turn bright green.

Transfer the hot vegetables to the bowl with the marinade and toss to coat. Marinate for at least 1 hour to allow the flavors to develop.

Serve the vegetables with a boiled rice.

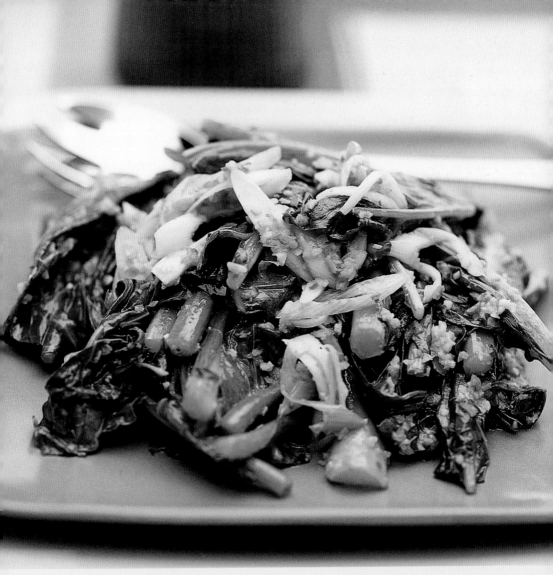

TRY THIS TASTY DISH,
COMBINING THE NUTRITIOUS
GOODNESS OF GREENS WITH
THE FLAVOR BURST OF CHILI
AND FRESH COCONUT.

nutrition per serving: Energy 223 Cal
Fat 19.8 g
Saturated fat 4.3 g
Protein 4.1 g
Carbohydrate 5.2 g
Fiber 5.1 g
Cholesterol 0 mg
Sodium 265 mg

PASTA SIRACUSA

This Mediterranean-style dish is a good source of antioxidants. If you're watching your weight use wholemeal spaghetti because it is more filling than white pasta.

2 tsp olive oil

2 garlic cloves, crushed

1 large green pepper, thinly sliced

28 oz canned reduced-salt diced tomatoes

2 zucchini, chopped

2 anchovy fillets in brine, drained
   and chopped

1 tbsp capers, chopped

3 tbsp black olives in brine, rinsed, pitted
   and halved

2 tbsp chopped basil

16 oz spaghetti or linguine

2/3 cup grated parmesan cheese, to serve

Prep time: 20 minutes

Cooking time: 30 minutes

Servings: 4–6

Heat the oil in a large, deep frying pan and cook the garlic for 30 seconds over low heat. Add the pepper, tomatoes, zucchini, anchovies, capers, olives and 1/2 cup water. Cook for 20 minutes, stirring occasionally.

Add the basil to the pan and stir well. Season to taste with freshly ground black pepper.

Meanwhile, cook the pasta in a large saucepan of boiling water for 10 minutes, or until *al dente.* Drain well. Serve the pasta topped with the sauce and grated parmesan.

nutrition per serving (6): Energy 394 Cal; Fat 6.5 g; Saturated fat 2.7 g; Protein 15.7 g; Carbohydrate 64.5 g; Fiber 5.4 g; Cholesterol 11 mg; Sodium 260 mg

SPINACH SHELLS IN TOMATO SAUCE

THIS LOW-FAT MEAL IS SUITABLE FOR VEGETARIANS WHO EAT DAIRY PRODUCTS AND IT PROVIDES GOOD AMOUNTS OF CALCIUM, B-GROUP VITAMINS AND ANTIOXIDANTS.

7 oz large pasta shells

9 oz frozen leaf spinach, defrosted

2 cups low-fat, reduced-salt cottage cheese

1 cup low-fat ricotta cheese

2 spring onions (scallions), finely chopped

1 tsp nutmeg

17 fl oz reduced-salt puréed tomatoes

1 cup reduced-salt vegetable stock or water

½ cup grated reduced-fat cheddar cheese (we used 50% reduced-fat)

PREP TIME: 20 MINUTES

COOKING TIME: 55 MINUTES

SERVINGS: 4–6

Cook the pasta in a large saucepan of boiling salted water for 10 minutes, or until *al dente*. Drain and cool under cold water.

Using clean hands, squeeze the excess moisture from the spinach. Put in a large bowl, add the cottage and ricotta cheeses, spring onions and nutmeg. Season well with freshly ground black pepper. Combine well using a fork.

Preheat the oven to 350°F. Combine half the pureed tomato and half the stock or water and pour over the base of a 9 x 13 in ovenproof dish. Spoon the spinach mixture into the pasta shells and put them in a single layer over the sauce. Spread over the remaining puréed tomatoes and stock or water and sprinkle over the cheese mixture.

Bake for 45 minutes, or until the pasta is cooked. Serve hot with a mixed green salad.

HINT:
• This meal can be prepared in advance.

nutrition per serving (6): Energy 316 Cal; Fat 5.8 g; Saturated fat 2.7 g; Protein 26.1 g; Carbohydrate 37.6 g; Fiber 4.9 g; Cholesterol 18 mg; Sodium 568 mg

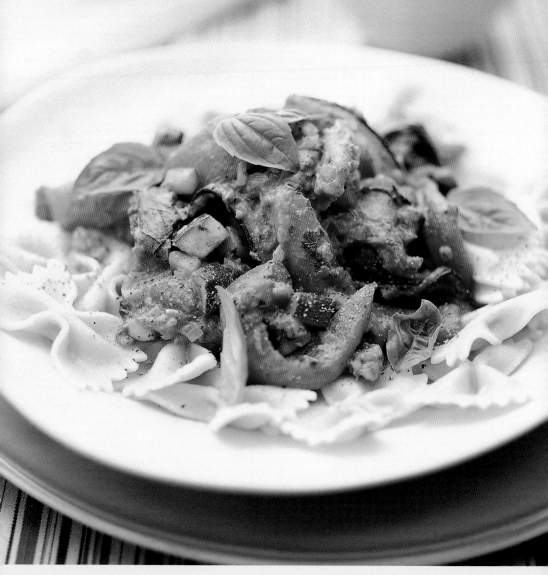

RATATOUILLE IS A VERSATILE
DISH THAT CAN BE SERVED
WITH RICE, POTATOES OR AS
A SIDE. HERE IT IS SERVED
ACCOMPANIED BY PASTA AS A
COMPLETE VEGETARIAN MEAL.

nutrition per serving: Energy 385 Cal
Fat 5.4 g
Saturated fat 1.8 g
Protein 12.6 g
Carbohydrate 65.5 g
Fiber 6.8 g
Cholesterol 11 mg
Sodium 31 mg

CREAMY RATATOUILLE WITH FARFALLE

1 to 2 baby eggplants
olive oil spray
1 large red pepper
1 large green pepper
2 tsp olive oil
1 onion, diced
4 garlic cloves, crushed
15 oz canned reduced-salt diced tomatoes
2 zucchini, finely diced
1 tbsp chopped thyme
3 tbsp chopped parsley
3 tbsp red wine
2 tsp brown sugar

2 tsp no-added-salt tomato paste
2½ handfuls basil, plus extra whole leaves, to serve
16 oz farfalle pasta
½ cup light cream

PREP TIME: 30 MINUTES
COOKING TIME: 55 MINUTES
SERVINGS: 6

Heat the grill or broiler to high. Cut the ends off the eggplants and slice the flesh lengthways into ¾ in strips. Spread the eggplant on a baking tray lined with foil and lightly spray with spray oil. Grill for about 3–5 minutes, or until golden brown, then remove.

Cut the peppers into large flat pieces and remove the seeds and membranes. Cook, skin side up, on the hot grill until the skin blackens and blisters. Leave to cool in a plastic bag, then peel away the skin and cut the flesh into strips.

Heat the oil in a large frying pan. Add the onion and garlic and gently sauté for 3 minutes. Stir through the grilled eggplant, pepper, tomato, zucchini, thyme, parsley, wine, sugar, tomato paste and basil. Season well with freshly ground pepper, then simmer, uncovered, for 30 minutes, stirring occasionally.

While the ratatouille is simmering, cook the pasta in a large saucepan of rapidly boiling, salted water for 10 minutes, or until *al dente*. Drain well and keep warm.

Take the ratatouille off the heat, add the cream and stir through gently. Divide the pasta among six serving bowls and spoon the ratatouille over the top. Garnish with the extra basil leaves and serve.

149

RED LENTIL AND RICOTTA LASAGNA

THIS LOW GI LASAGNA IS AN EXCELLENT CHOICE FOR VEGETARIANS. IT PROVIDES GOOD AMOUNTS OF COMPLETE PROTEIN, CALCIUM AND ANTIOXIDANTS.

½ cup red lentils

2 tsp olive oil

2–3 garlic cloves, crushed

1 large onion, chopped

1 small red pepper, chopped

2 zucchini, sliced

1 celery stalk, sliced

28 oz canned reduced-salt diced tomatoes

2 tbsp no-added-salt tomato paste

1 tsp dried oregano

⅓ cup cornstarch

3 cups skim milk

¼ onion

½ tsp ground nutmeg

1⅓ cups low-fat ricotta cheese

12 dried or fresh lasagna sheets

½ cup grated reduced-fat cheddar cheese

PREP TIME: 30 MINUTES + 30 MINUTES
  SOAKING

COOKING TIME: 1 HOUR 50 MINUTES

SERVINGS: 6

Pour the lentils in a large bowl, cover with boiling water and soak for 30 minutes. Drain. Heat the oil in a large saucepan, add the garlic and onion and cook for 2 minutes. Add the pepper, zucchini and celery and cook for 2–3 minutes, or until softened. Add the lentils, tomatoes, tomato paste, oregano and 1½ cups water. Bring slowly to a boil, then reduce the heat and simmer for 30 minutes, or until the lentils are tender. Stir occasionally. Preheat the oven to 350°F.

To make the white sauce, blend the cornstarch with 2 tablespoons of the milk in a saucepan until smooth. Pour the remaining milk into the pan, add the onion and stir over low heat until the mixture boils and thickens. Add the nutmeg and season with freshly ground black pepper, then cook over low heat for 5 minutes. Remove the onion.

Beat the ricotta with about ½ cup of the white sauce. Spread one-third of the lentil mixture over the base of a 9 x 13 in ovenproof dish. Cover with a layer of lasagna sheets. Spread another third of the lentil mixture over the pasta, then spread the ricotta mixture evenly over the top. Follow with another layer of lasagna, then the remaining lentils. Pour the white sauce over the top. Sprinkle with the grated cheese. Bake for 1 hour, covering with lightly oiled foil if the top starts to brown too much. Stand for 5 minutes before cutting. Serve with a salad.

nutrition per serving: Energy 398 Cal; Fat 7.9 g; Saturated fat 2.9 g; Protein 23.7 g; Carbohydrate 55.4 g; Fiber 6.9 g; Cholesterol 10 mg; Sodium 232 mg

SPICY VEGETABLE STEW WITH DHAL

THIS INDIAN-STYLE DISH COMBINES THE GOODNESS OF FRESH VEGETABLES AND LEGUMES, PROVIDING A NOURISHING AND FILLING MEAL. IT IS LOW IN FAT, CHOLESTEROL-FREE, AND A GOOD SOURCE OF FOLATE AND POTASSIUM.

DHAL
¾ cup yellow split peas
2 in piece of ginger, grated
2–3 garlic cloves, crushed
1 red chili, seeded and chopped

3 tomatoes
1 tbsp oil
1 tsp yellow mustard seeds
1 tsp cumin seeds
1 tsp ground cumin
½ tsp garam masala
1 red onion, cut into thin wedges

3 slender eggplants, thickly sliced
2 carrots, thickly sliced
¼ cauliflower, cut into florets
1½ cups reduced-salt vegetable stock
2 small zucchini, thickly sliced
½ cup frozen peas
½ cup fresh cilantro leaves

PREP TIME: 25 MINUTES + 2 HOURS SOAKING
COOKING TIME: 1 HOUR 35 MINUTES
SERVINGS: 4–6

To make the dhal, put the split peas in a bowl, cover with water and soak for 2 hours. Drain. Place in a large saucepan with the ginger, garlic, chili and 3 cups water. Bring to a boil, reduce the heat and simmer for 45 minutes, or until soft.

Score a cross in the base of each tomato, soak in boiling water for 30 seconds, then plunge into cold water and peel the skin away from the cross. Seed and thoroughly chop.

Heat the oil in a large saucepan. Cook the spices over medium heat for 30 seconds, or until fragrant. Add the onion and cook for 2 minutes, or until the onion is soft. Stir in the tomato, eggplant, carrot and cauliflower.

Add the dhal and stock, mix together well and simmer, covered, for 45 minutes, or until the vegetables are tender. Stir occasionally. Add the zucchini and peas during the last 10 minutes of cooking. Stir in the cilantro leaves and serve.

nutrition per serving (6): Energy 178 Cal; Fat 4.5 g; Saturated fat 0.4 g; Protein 10 g; Carbohydrate 21.2 g; Fiber 7.3 g; Cholesterol 0 mg; Sodium 282 mg

151

CARAMELIZED ONIONS AND LENTILS WITH ENGLISH SPINACH

¼ cups lentils
1 tbsp olive oil
2 red onions, finely sliced
2 garlic cloves, finely chopped
1 tsp ground coriander
1 tsp ground cumin
about 1 lb English spinach, rinsed well and
  stems trimmed
1 tbsp lemon juice

2 tbsp chopped cilantro leaves

PREP TIME: 20 MINUTES
COOKING TIME: 1 HOUR
SERVINGS: 6

Put the lentils in a small saucepan over high heat and add 2½ cups water. Bring to a boil, then cover with a fitted lid, reduce the heat to very low and simmer the lentils for 35 minutes, or until all of the water has been absorbed and the lentils are tender.

Meanwhile, heat the oil in a frying pan over medium heat and cook the onion, stirring occasionally, for 20 minutes, or until soft and caramelized. Add the garlic, ground coriander and cumin, season with freshly ground black pepper and cook for a further 3 minutes. Remove from the heat.

Put the spinach in a large steamer and cover with a lid. Sit the steamer over a saucepan or wok of boiling water and steam for 3–5 minutes, or until wilted. Combine the lentils, onion mixture and spinach in a large bowl, add the lemon juice and cilantro and toss well. Serve immediately.

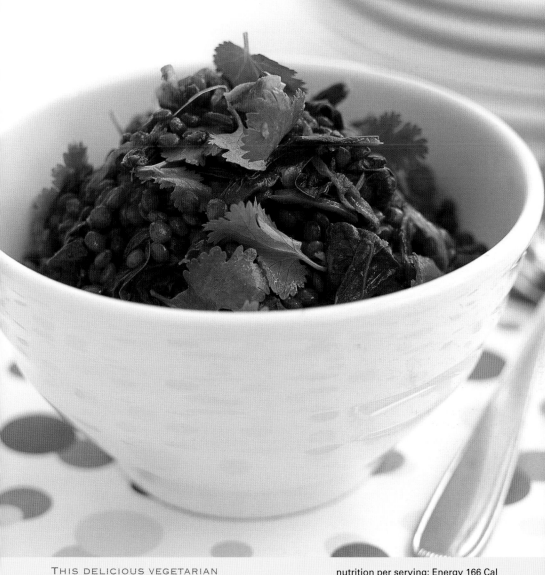

THIS DELICIOUS VEGETARIAN
DISH IS LOW-GI, HIGH IN FIBER
AND A GOOD SOURCE OF
FOLATE AND ANTIOXIDANTS.

nutrition per serving: Energy 166 Cal
Fat 4.2 g
Saturated fat 0.6 g
Protein 11.8 g
Carbohydrate 16.9 g
Fiber 8.2 g
Cholesterol 0 mg
Sodium 25 mg

SPINACH PIE

YOU CAN STILL ENJOY DELICIOUS PIES, IN MODERATION, ON A LOW-FAT DIET—
JUST MAKE SURE THEY'RE MADE WITH FILO PASTRY AND LOW-FAT FILLINGS.

olive or canola oil spray
about 3 lbs English spinach, trimmed and
   washed
2 tsp olive oil
1 onion, chopped
4 spring onions, chopped
2¾ cups low-fat cottage cheese
2 eggs, lightly beaten
2 garlic cloves, crushed
pinch of ground nutmeg

¼ cup chopped mint
8 sheets filo pastry
½ cup fresh breadcrumbs

PREP TIME: 25 MINUTES
COOKING TIME: 50 MINUTES
SERVINGS: 6

Preheat the oven to 350°F. Lightly spray a 9 in square x 2 in deep ovenproof dish with oil.
Place the spinach in a large pan. Cover and cook for 2–3 minutes, or until just wilted.
Drain, cool, then squeeze dry and chop.

Heat the oil in a small frying pan. Cook the onion and spring onion for 2–3 minutes, or until
softened. Combine with the spinach. Stir in the cheese, egg, garlic, nutmeg and mint.
Season with freshly ground black pepper, and mix thoroughly.

Spray a sheet of filo pastry with spray oil. Fold in half widthways and line the base and
sides of the dish. Repeat with three more sheets. Keep the unused sheets moist by
covering with a damp dish towel.

Sprinkle the breadcrumbs over the pastry. Spread the filling in the dish. Fold over any
overlapping pastry. Spray and fold another sheet and place on top. Repeat with three
more sheets. Tuck the pastry in. Spray the top with more oil. Score squares on top. Bake
for 40 minutes, or until golden.

nutrition per serving: Energy 295 Cal; Fat 7.1 g; Saturated fat 2 g; Protein 33.2 g; Carbohydrate 20.2
g; Fiber 7.9 g; Cholesterol 79 mg; Sodium 416 mg

BAKED VEGETABLES WITH GARLIC AND ROSEMARY

WITH LESS FAT THAN REGULAR ROAST VEGETABLES, THIS HEALTHY COMBINATION PROVIDES CARBOHYDRATE ENERGY, FIBER, BETA-CAROTENE, FOLATE AND POTASSIUM.

2 carrots

2 parsnips

2 large potatoes

1 medium pumpkin or winter squash

olive oil spray

2 slender eggplants

4 large garlic cloves, unpeeled

4 small sprigs of rosemary

2 tbsp chopped parsley

PREP TIME: 15 MINUTES

COOKING TIME: 40 MINUTES

SERVINGS: 4

Preheat the oven to 400°F. Wash the vegetables and pat dry. Cut the carrots and parsnips in half lengthways, then crossways. Quarter the potatoes. Cut the unpeeled pumpkin into chunks.

Put the carrot, parsnip, potato and pumpkin in a baking dish and spray lightly with oil. Sprinkle with freshly ground black pepper. Bake for 20 minutes, turning occasionally.

Meanwhile, cut the eggplants in half lengthways and make thin shallow cuts through the skin. Add to the baking dish with the garlic and rosemary sprigs. Spray with more oil and cook, turning occasionally, for 20 minutes, or until all of the vegetables are tender. To serve, squeeze out the soft garlic and serve with the vegetables and the rosemary. Sprinkle with the parsley and more freshly ground black pepper.

nutrition per serving: Energy 153 Cal; Fat 1.9 g; Saturated fat 0.4 g; Protein 5.4 g; Carbohydrate 24.8 g; Fiber 6 g; Cholesterol 0 mg; Sodium 30 mg

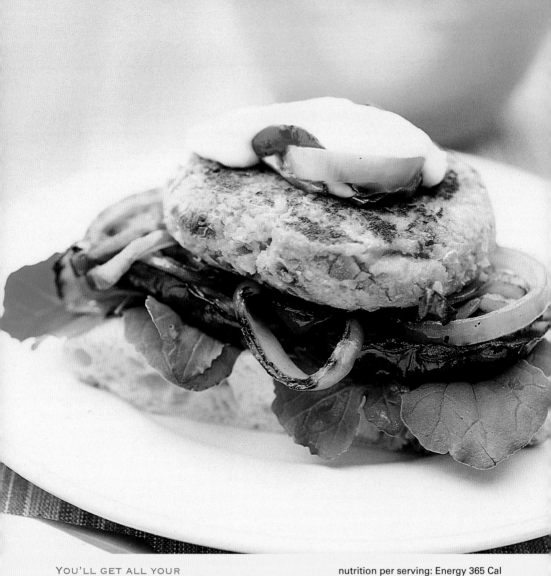

You'll get all your nutrients in one hit with this spicy vegetarian burger. Much better than takeout and tastier too!

nutrition per serving: Energy 365 Cal
Fat 6.1 g
Saturated fat 1.2 g
Protein 15.3 g
Carbohydrate 56.6 g
Fiber 9.2 g
Cholesterol 3 mg
Sodium 395 mg

CHICKPEA BURGERS

CHICKPEA PATTIES
2 tsp olive oil
1 small onion, finely chopped
2 garlic cloves, crushed
28 oz canned chickpeas, drained
  and rinsed
½ cup cooked brown rice
⅓ cup sun-dried tomatoes, chopped

1 eggplant, cut into ½ in slices
1 large red onion, sliced into rings
spray olive oil
2 large handfuls arugula leaves
6 pieces pita bread

SPICY YOGURT DRESSING
7 oz reduced-fat plain yogurt
1 garlic clove, crushed
¼ tsp ground cumin
¼ tsp ground coriander

PREP TIME: 30 MINUTES + 1 HOUR
  REFRIGERATION
COOKING TIME: 20 MINUTES
MAKES 6 BURGERS

To make the chickpea patties, heat the oil in a frying pan and cook the onion over medium heat for 2 minutes, or until soft and lightly golden. Add the garlic and cook for 1 more minute, then remove from the heat and allow to cool slightly. Put the onion mixture in a food processor or blender with the chickpeas, rice and sun-dried tomato. Using a pulse action, process in short bursts until the mixture is combined and the chickpeas are broken up, but not completely mushy, scraping the bowl down with a spatula a few times during processing. Season with freshly ground black pepper, then shape the mixture into six patties about 3¼ in in diameter. Place on a tray lined with plastic wrap, then cover and refrigerate for 1 hour.

Put all the spicy yogurt dressing ingredients in a small bowl and mix together well. Refrigerate until needed.

Preheat a cast-iron or nonstick skillet to moderately hot. Spray the eggplant slices and onion rings lightly on each side with spray oil. Cook the eggplant and onion until tender and lightly golden—the eggplant will need about 3–4 minutes each side, the onion about 5 minutes. Transfer the vegetables to a plate and set aside.

Spray the top of the chickpea patties lightly with oil, then put them face-down on the pan and cook for 3 minutes. Spray the top of the patties with a little more oil, then turn and cook for a further 3 minutes, or until golden.

While the chickpea patties are cooking, arrange the arugula, eggplant and onion on the pita bread. Add the hot chickpea patties, dollop with some of the spicy yogurt dressing and serve at once.

VEGETABLE FRITTATA

A NOURISHING SNACK OR MEAL WITH MORE NUTRIENTS THAN SCRAMBLED EGGS, THIS DISH IS A GOOD SOURCE OF VITAMIN A, FOLATE, VITAMIN B12 AND HIGH-QUALITY PROTEIN.

1 large zucchini, cubed
1 small pumpkin or winter squash, cubed
1 large potato, cubed
½ cup broccoli florets
2 tsp olive oil
1 small onion, chopped
1 small red pepper, chopped
2 tbsp finely chopped fresh parsley

olive oil spray
3 eggs
2 egg whites
mixed-leaf salad, to serve

PREP TIME: 25 MINUTES
COOKING TIME: 25 MINUTES
SERVINGS: 6

Steam the zucchini, pumpkin, potato and broccoli until tender, then transfer to a bowl.

Heat the oil in a non-stick frying pan, about 9 in in diameter. Add the onion and pepper, and cook for 3 minutes, or until tender. Transfer to the bowl of steamed vegetables, along with the chopped parsley.

Heat a frying pan over medium heat and spray with oil. Return all the vegetables to the pan and spread out with a spatula to an even thickness. Beat the eggs and egg whites together and pour into the pan, tilting to distribute evenly.

Cook over medium heat until the egg is almost set, but still runny on top. Wrap the handle of the pan in a damp dish towel to protect it and place the pan under the grill to cook the frittata top (pierce gently with a fork to make sure it is cooked through). Cut into wedges and serve.

nutrition per serving: Energy 129 Cal; Fat 5.2 g; Saturated fat 1.2 g; Protein 8 g; Carbohydrate 11.1 g; Fiber 3 g; Cholesterol 94 mg; Sodium 59 mg

SWISS CHARD PARCELS

A DELICIOUS BLEND OF RISOTTO, CHEESE AND VEGETABLES IN NUTRITIOUS SWISS CHARD DELIVERS CARBOHYDRATE, B-GROUP VITAMINS, FOLATE, VITAMIN C AND POTASSIUM.

2 cups reduced-salt vegetable stock
2 tsp olive oil
1 onion, chopped
2 garlic cloves, crushed
½ cup arborio rice
1 red pepper, chopped
9 oz mushrooms, chopped
½ cup grated reduced-fat cheddar cheese
¼ cup shredded fresh basil
6 large swiss chard leaves

28 oz canned reduced-salt diced tomatoes
1 tbsp balsamic vinegar
1 tsp soft brown sugar

PREP TIME: 40 MINUTES
COOKING TIME: 1 HOUR
SERVINGS: 6

Heat the stock in a pan and maintain at simmering point. Heat the oil in a large pan, add the onion and garlic and cook until softened. Add the rice, pepper and mushrooms, and stir until well combined. Gradually add ½ cup hot stock, stirring until the liquid is absorbed. Add the stock, a little at a time, stirring until it is all absorbed and the rice is tender (about 20 minutes). Remove from the heat, add the cheese and basil, and season well with freshly ground black pepper.

Meanwhile, trim the stalks from the swiss chard and cook the leaves, a few at a time, in a large pan of boiling water for 30 seconds, or until wilted. Drain on a dish towel. Cut away any tough veins from the leaves. Put a portion of risotto filling in the center of each leaf, fold in the sides and roll up carefully. Tie with string.

Put the tomato, vinegar and sugar in a large, deep non-stick frying pan and stir to combine. Add the swiss chard parcels, cover and simmer for 10 minutes. Remove the string and serve with tomato sauce.

nutrition per serving: Energy 187 Cal; Fat 4.5 g; Saturated fat 1.6 g; Protein 9 g; Carbohydrate 24.2 g; Fiber 6.1 g; Cholesterol 6 mg; Sodium 420 mg

SWEET POTATO STRUDEL

1 large sweet potato, cut into ¾ in cubes

3 garlic cloves, unpeeled

olive oil spray

9 oz spinach, blanched and excess
   moisture squeezed out, roughly chopped

¼ cup pine nuts, toasted

4½ oz low-fat feta cheese, crumbled

3 spring onions (scallions), including green
   part, chopped

2 tbsp black olives, pitted and sliced

¼ cup chopped basil

1 tbsp chopped rosemary

8 sheets filo pastry

1 tbsp sesame seeds

PREP TIME: 25 MINUTES

COOKING TIME: 1 HOUR 5 MINUTES

SERVINGS: 6

Preheat the oven to moderate 350°F. Put the sweet potato and garlic in a roasting pan and spray with oil. Roast for 30 minutes, or until the sweet potato is soft. Remove the garlic when it is soft, after about 15 minutes. Cool slightly.

Combine the sweet potato, spinach, pine nuts, feta, spring onion, olives, basil and rosemary. Peel the garlic cloves and roughly chop the flesh, then add to the sweet potato mixture, and season with freshly ground black pepper.

Cover the pastry with a damp dish towel to prevent it drying out. Lay the pastry out in front of you, in a stack, and spray each layer with oil. Spread the filling in the center of the pastry, covering an area 4 x 12 in. Fold in the shorter ends of the pastry. Fold the long side closest to you over the filling, then carefully roll up. Place the strudel on a greased baking tray, seam side down. Spray with oil and sprinkle with sesame seeds. Bake for 35 minutes, or until crisp and golden. Serve warm.

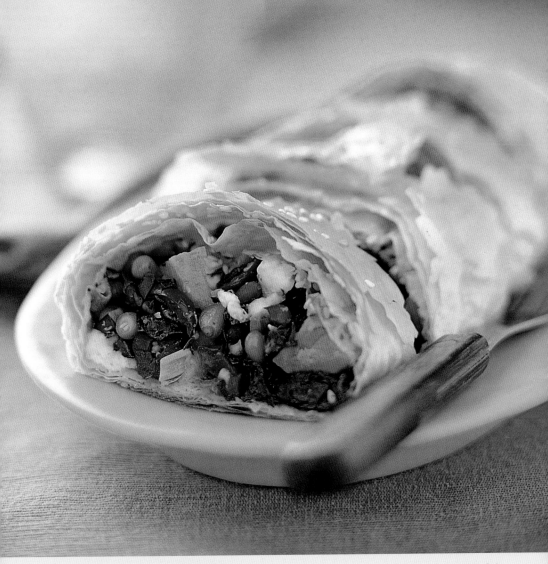

THIS TASTY AND COLORFUL DISH
IS GREAT TO SERVE TO FRIENDS.
THE VARIETY OF INGREDIENTS
DELIVERS GOOD AMOUNTS
OF MONOUNSATURATED FAT
AND FIBER.

nutrition per serving: Energy 221 Cal
Fat 10.9 g
Saturated fat 2.6 g
Protein 9.9 g
Carbohydrate 19.1 g
Fiber 3.6 g
Cholesterol 4 mg
Sodium 436 mg

SWEET THINGS

MANGO PASSIONFRUIT SORBET

CLEBRATE THE SUMMER MONTHS WITH THIS TASTY SORBET. IT CONTAINS GOOD AMOUNTS OF FIBER AND ANTIOXIDANTS.

1 cup sugar
⅓ cup passionfruit pulp (about 8 passionfruit)
½ large mango, chopped
1 large peach, chopped
2 tbsp lemon juice
1 egg white

PREP TIME: 20 MINUTES + REFRIGERATION TIME + 8 HOURS FREEZING
COOKING TIME: 5 MINUTES
SERVINGS: 6

Put the sugar in a saucepan with 1 cup water. Stir over low heat until the sugar has dissolved. Increase the heat, bring to a boil and boil for 1 minute. Transfer to a glass bowl, cool, then refrigerate. Strain the passionfruit pulp, reserving 1 tablespoon of the seeds.

Blend the fruit, passionfruit juice and lemon juice in a blender until smooth. With the motor running, add the cold sugar syrup and ½ cup + 2 tbsp water. Stir in the passionfruit seeds. Freeze in a shallow container, stirring occasionally, for about 5 hours, or until almost set.

Break up the icy mixture roughly with a fork or spoon, transfer to a bowl and beat with electric beaters until smooth and fluffy. Beat the egg white in a small bowl until firm peaks form, then fold into the mixture until just combined. Spread into a loaf pan and return to the freezer until firm. Transfer to the refrigerator, to soften, 15 minutes before serving.

HINT:
• To make a berry sorbet, use 1 cup blackberries or blueberries, 1 cup hulled strawberries and ¼ cup peach flesh. Prepare as above.

nutrition per serving: Energy 188 Cal; Fat 0.1 g; Saturated fat 0 g; Protein 1.6 g; Carbohydrate 44.7 g; Fiber 3 g; Cholesterol 0 mg; Sodium 13 mg

PEAR SORBET

THIS FRESH FRUIT SORBET IS MADE WITH SUCRALOSE INSTEAD OF SUGAR
SO IT'S GOOD IF YOU ARE WATCHING YOUR WEIGHT OR HAVE DIABETES.

6 large very ripe pears
1 cup sucralose

PREP TIME: 40 MINUTES + OVERNIGHT
FREEZING
COOKING TIME: 15 MINUTES
SERVINGS: 4–6

Thickly peel the pears, then core them and slice them into thick pieces. Place the pears in
a large saucepan, just cover with water and simmer for about 10 minutes, or until tender.
Drain and allow to cool.

Purée the pears in a blender or food processor until smooth.

Combine the sucralose and ¾ cup + 2 tbsp water in a saucepan over medium heat. Allow
the syrup to cool. Mix together the sucralose syrup and pear purée, then pour into a
shallow metal pan. Freeze until just solid.

Remove the pan from the freezer. Beat or process until a "slush" forms. Return to the pan
and freeze until firm. Remove from freezer 15–20 minutes before serving.

HINT:
• Sorbets may be served before the main course to refresh the palate, or with other
  creams or fruit as a dessert.

nutrition per serving: Energy 130 Cal; Fat 0.2 g; Saturated fat 0 g; Protein 0.6 g; Carbohydrate 30.8 g;
Fiber 3.7 g; Cholesterol 0 mg; Sodium 7 mg

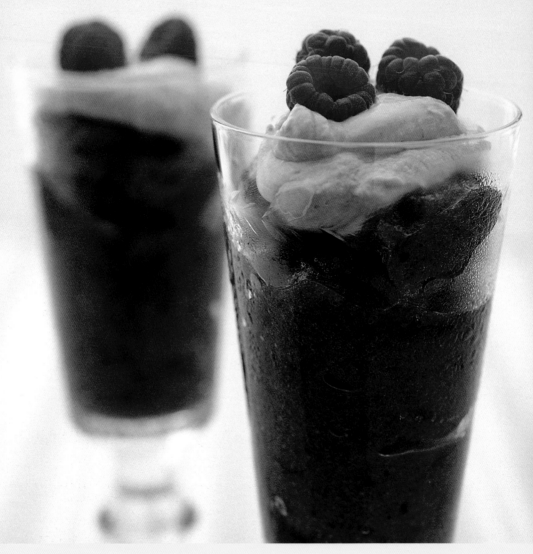

DAZZLE YOUR FRIENDS
WITH THIS DELICIOUS SUNDAE.
IT'S LOW GI AND CALORIES,
AND BERRIES ARE PROVIDES
GOOD AMOUNTS OF FIBER
AND ANTIOXIDANTS.

nutrition per serving: Energy 95 Cal
Fat 1.7 g
Saturated fat 1 g
Protein 2.6 g
Carbohydrate 14.9 g
Fiber 3.9 g
Cholesterol 8 mg
Sodium 17 mg

166

MIXED BERRY SUNDAE WITH RASPBERRY CREAM

1¾ oz sucralose
juice of 1 lemon
about 2 lbs mixed summer berries,
    including blueberries, raspberries and
    strawberries
extra fresh berries, to serve

RASPBERRY CREAM
2 cups fresh raspberries
½ cup confectioners' sugar
½ cup whipping cream

PREP TIME: 15 MINUTES + 7 HOURS
    FREEZING
COOKING TIME: NONE
SERVINGS: 10

Put 2 cups water in a saucepan and add the sucralose. Heat gently over low heat until the sucralose has dissolved. Bring to a boil, then reduce the heat and simmer for 5 minutes. Set aside to cool, then stir in the lemon juice.

Put the sweet syrup and mixed berries in a large processor fitted with the metal blade and blend for 20 seconds, or until smooth. Press the purée through a sieve in batches and pour into a wide, deep plastic container.

Freeze the mixture for 1–2 hours, or until ice crystals have formed around the edges. Using an immersion blender or blender, blend to break up the ice crystals. Return to the freezer and repeat this process for 4–5 hours until the berry mixture resembles soft snow. Remove from freezer 15–20 minutes before serving.

To make the raspberry cream, blend the raspberries and confectioners' sugar in a small processor for 10 seconds, or until smooth. Press through a fine sieve. Lightly whip the cream until it just holds its shape. Fold the cream into the raspberry purée.

Serve the frozen sundae mixture in chilled glasses with a spoonful of raspberry cream and some fresh berries.

STEWED PEAR, APPLE AND RHUBARB WITH CUSTARD

A HEALTHY, LOW FAT TREAT FOR THE WHOLE FAMILY, THIS DESSERT IS LOADED WITH POTASSIUM, MANGANESE AND CALCIUM.

2 tbsp blackcurrant syrup

2 large pears, peeled, cored and quartered

1 apple, peeled, cored and quartered

about 1 lb rhubarb, trimmed, cut into 1¼ in pieces

2 cups skim milk

¼ cup sugar

1½ tbsp custard powder or instant vanilla pudding mix

PREP TIME: 20 MINUTES

COOKING TIME: 20 MINUTES

SERVINGS: 4

Put the syrup, pears, apple and ¼ cup water in a large saucepan and stir to coat the fruits. Cook, covered, over low heat for 4 minutes, then add the rhubarb. Toss well to combine, then cover and cook for a further 6–7 minutes, or until the fruit is just tender. Remove from the heat, cover and leave to stand.

Put the milk and sugar in a saucepan. Bring to a boil, then reduce the heat and simmer for 3 minutes. Mix the custard powder with 1 tablespoon water to a smooth paste. Return the milk to a boil, stir in the custard powder mixture and whisk constantly until the mixture boils and thickens, and can coat the back of a wooden spoon.

Put the fruit in serving dishes and drizzle with any liquid from the bottom of the pan. Serve with the warm custard.

nutrition per serving: Energy 231 Cal; Fat 0.4 g; Saturated fat 0.2 g; Protein 5.8 g; Carbohydrate 50.5 g; Fiber 4 g; Cholesterol 4 mg; Sodium 65 mg

PEACH YOGURT MOUSSE

THIS LIGHT DESSERT IS GREAT IN SUMMER WHEN PEACHES ARE IN SEASON. IT'S HIGH IN POTASSIUM AND PROVIDES SOME FIBER AND CALCIUM.

1 cup dried peaches

1 cup peach nectar

2 tsp powdered gelatin

¾ cup reduced-fat plain yogurt

2–3 tsp honey, to taste

3 egg whites

2 tbsp toasted flaked almonds, to serve

PREP TIME: 15 MINUTES + 1 HOUR REFRIGERATION

COOKING TIME: 10 MINUTES

SERVINGS: 4

Put the peaches and peach nectar in a small saucepan. Cook over low heat, stirring often, for 10 minutes, or until the peaches are soft and pulpy. Set aside to cool for 10 minutes.

Put 2 tablespoons of hot water in a small bowl and sprinkle the gelatin over the top. Whisk with a fork for 1 minute, or until the gelatin has dissolved.

Put the peach mixture, gelatin mixture and yogurt in a small processor or blender fitted with the metal blade. Process for 20–30 seconds, or until smooth. Add the honey, to taste, and blend to combine.

Whisk the egg whites until firm peaks form. Pour the peach mixture into the egg whites and gently fold through using a metal spoon.

Spoon the mousse into 1 cup parfait glasses and smooth the surface. Cover and refrigerate for at least 1 hour, or until firm. Serve sprinkled with the almonds.

nutrition per serving: Energy 205 Cal; Fat 4.6 g; Saturated fat 0.8 g; Protein 9.7 g; Carbohydrate 29.2 g; Fiber 3.3 g; Cholesterol 5 mg; Sodium 84 mg

STICKY FIG AND HAZELNUT PUDDINGS

⅓ cup hazelnuts
1 cup + 1 tbsp fresh orange juice
½ cup chopped dried figs, plus 6 dried figs,
   extra, cut horizontally
¼ tsp ground ginger
¼ tsp ground cinnamon
3 tsp finely grated orange zest
½ tsp baking soda
½ cup canola margarine, softened
½ cup brown sugar

1 egg
¾ cup self-rising flour
2 tbsp maple syrup
boiling water, for steaming
low-fat vanilla custard or cream, to serve

PREP TIME: 25 MINUTES + 10 MINUTES
   COOLING TIME
COOKING TIME: 45 MINUTES
MAKES 6

Preheat the oven to 400°F. Spread the hazelnuts out on a tray and place in the oven for 6–7 minutes, until lightly toasted. Tip the nuts onto a clean dish towel and gently rub to remove the skins. Put the nuts in a food processor and pulse until finely ground. Grease 6 x 1 cup ramekins or ovenproof teacups and place a square of baking paper in the base of each.

Pour the orange juice into a saucepan and bring to a boil over medium heat. Add the chopped figs, ginger, cinnamon and 1 teaspoon of the orange zest and cook for 1 minute. Remove from the heat and add the baking soda (allowing the mixture to froth), then set aside to cool for 10 minutes.

Meanwhile, combine the margarine and sugar in a large bowl and beat with electric beaters until light and fluffy. Add the egg and beat until well combined. Fold in the hazelnuts, and add the flour in three batches, incorporating each batch well into the mixture before adding the next (the mixture will become stiff). Pour the orange sauce into the pudding mixture and stir well to combine.

Pour the maple syrup into the base of the ramekins and top with the remaining orange zest. Arrange two of the extra fig halves in the base of each ramekin. Spoon in the pudding mixture until each ramikin is three-quarters full, then cover securely with a square sheet of foil. Arrange the puddings in the base of a deep roasting tin. Fill the baking tin with enough boiling water to come halfway up the sides of the ramekins, and bake the puddings for 35 minutes, or until cooked. Set the ramekins aside for 5 minutes before inverting onto a plate and serving with custard or cream.

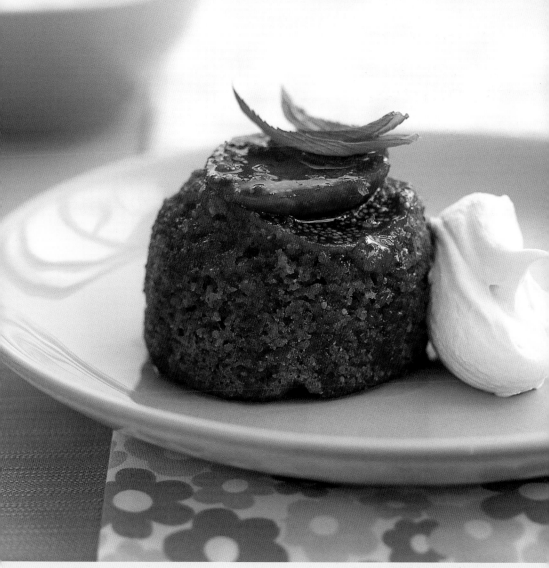

THIS RECIPE IS A LOWER FAT
VERSION OF STICKY DATE
PUDDING, BUT ENJOY IN
MODERATION—IT'S NOT LOW
IN CALORIES.

nutrition per serving: Energy 465 Cal
Fat 14.2 g
Saturated fat 2.4 g
Protein 9.5 g
Carbohydrate 74 g
Fiber 6.6 g
Cholesterol 38 mg
Sodium 406 mg

171

COUSCOUS AND APRICOT PUDDINGS

A GOOD CHOICE FOR PEOPLE WITH HIGH BLOOD PRESSURE AS WELL AS HIGH CHOLESTEROL—THIS DESSET IS HIGH IN POTASSIUM AND LOW IN CHOLESTEROL.

½ cup dried apricots, chopped
3½ cups apricot nectar
1 tbsp grated lemon zest
1 vanilla bean, split, seeds scraped
1 cinnamon stick
¼ tsp ground cloves
1 tbsp lemon juice

1 cup couscous
low-fat vanilla custard, to serve

PREP TIME: 20 MINUTES
COOKING TIME: 45 MINUTES
SERVINGS: 6

Grease 6 x 1 cup pudding bowls or ovenproof teacups and put a round of baking paper in the bottom of each. Combine the apricots, nectar, lemon zest, vanilla bean and seeds, and cinnamon stick in a saucepan over medium heat and bring to a boil.

Reduce the heat and simmer for 5 minutes, then remove from the heat and leave for 5 minutes. Strain, reserving the apricots and discarding the vanilla bean and cinnamon stick. Return the nectar to the saucepan and divide the apricots among the pudding bowls.

Add the cloves, lemon juice and couscous to the reserved apricot nectar. Bring to a boil, then reduce the heat to low and simmer, covered, for 8–10 minutes, or until most of the liquid has been absorbed. The mixture should still be quite wet.

Spoon the couscous into the pudding bowls, level the top and cover each with a round of foil. Place the bowls in a steamer and cover with a lid. Sit the steamer over a saucepan or wok of boiling water and steam for 30 minutes, checking the water level regularly.

To serve, turn the puddings out of the bowls and serve hot with custard.

nutrition per serving: Energy 323 Cal; Fat 1.4 g; Saturated fat 0.8 g; Protein 9.4 g; Carbohydrate 67 g; Fiber 3.2 g; Cholesterol 7 mg; Sodium 69 mg

PEAR AND GINGER FILO PARCELS

THESE REDUCED-FAT PARCELS ARE A GREAT DESSERT TO SERVE AT A DINNER
PARTY. THE PEAR PROVIDES POTASSIUM AND SOLUBLE FIBER.

¼ cup raisins

1 tbsp cognac or pear eau-de-vie

2 tsp lemon juice

3 Bosc pears

¼ cup ginger snaps, roughly broken

¼ cup brown sugar

½ tsp pumpkin pie spice

2 tbsp cornstarch

1 egg yolk

8 sheets filo pastry

canola oil spray

confectioners' sugar, to serve

softened low-fat vanilla ice cream, to serve

PREP TIME: 30 MINUTES

COOKING TIME: 25 MINUTES

SERVINGS: 4

Preheat the oven to 375°F. Line a baking tray with baking paper.

Put the raisins and liqueur in a small bowl and set aside. Put the lemon juice in a bowl. Peel, quarter and core the pears. Add them to the bowl and toss to coat with the lemon juice.

Put the cookies in a mini processor or blender and add the sugar, mixed spice and cornstarch. Blend for 15 seconds, or until the mixture forms fine crumbs. Roughly chop half the pears and add to the processor. Add the egg yolk and blend in 2-second bursts for 15–25 seconds, or until the pears are chopped medium–fine. The mixture will be quite thin.

Cut the remaining pears into ¾ in dice and return to their bowl. Add the raisin mixture and processed pear mixture and toss to combine.

Lay a sheet of filo on a work surface and spray with oil. Fold in half, one short side over the other and spray with oil. Top with another sheet of filo, fold that in half and spray with oil, giving four layers of pastry. Trim the pastry to an 7 in square. Spoon one-quarter of the pear filling onto the center. Starting at one corner, fold the filo over the filling to make a fat, square envelope. Ensure that the filling is well contained, and spray dry surfaces of the pastry as you fold. Spray the parcel all over with oil and place on the prepared tray, fold side up. Make three more parcels using the remaining pastry and filling.

Bake for 20–25 minutes, or until the parcels are crisp and golden. Serve hot, dusted with confectioners' sugar and with a little softened vanilla ice cream spooned on top.

nutrition per serving: Energy 402 Cal; Fat 7.3 g; Saturated fat 2.4 g; Protein 6.9 g; Carbohydrate 75.8 g; Fiber 3.8 g; Cholesterol 51 mg; Sodium 291 mg

173

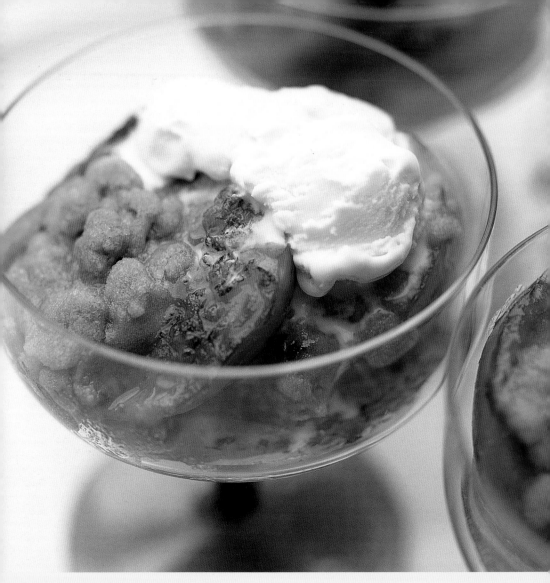

THIS TASTY DISH IS READY IN A FLASH. IT HAS LESS FAT THAN TRADITIONAL CRUMBLES, BUT STILL HAS ALL THE FLAVOR.

nutrition per serving: Energy 250 Cal
Fat 4.8 g
Saturated fat 1.5 g
Protein 4.7 g
Carbohydrate 46.1 g
Fiber 3.9 g
Cholesterol 5 mg
Sodium 91 mg

NECTARINE CRUMBLE WITH MAPLE AND LIME SYRUP

3 tbsp maple syrup
1 tsp finely grated lime zest
4 ripe nectarines, cut in half, pits removed
¼ cup self-rising flour
2 tbsp light canola margarine
2 tbsp brown sugar
low-fat vanilla ice cream, to serve

PREP TIME: 20 MINUTES + 15 MINUTES
INFUSING TIME
COOKING TIME: 5 MINUTES
SERVINGS: 4

Put the maple syrup and lime zest in a bowl. Stir well and leave to infuse for 15 minutes.

Heat the broiler to medium. Lightly brush the cut side of the nectarine halves with some of the syrup. Put the nectarine halves, cut side down, in a lightly oiled non-stick frying pan. Gently fry over low–medium heat for 1 minute on each side, or until slightly soft.

Put the flour in a small bowl and add the butter. Using your fingertips, rub the butter into the flour until the mixture resembles breadcrumbs, then stir through the sugar.

Sit the nectarines on a baking tray, cut side up. Lightly brush them with a little more syrup, then sprinkle the crumble mixture over the top and broil for 2 minutes, or until the crumble turns golden brown. Divide among four serving bowls and drizzle with the remaining syrup. Serve with a scoop of low-fat vanilla ice cream.

REDUCED-FAT CHOCOLATE CAKE WITH STRAWBERRIES

WHO CAN SAY NO TO A SLICE OF CHOCOLATE CAKE? THIS VERSION HAS LESS FAT THAN TRADITIONAL CHOCOLATE CAKES BUT SHOULD BE ENJOYED IN MODERATION.

3 eggs
1 cup lightly packed brown sugar
3 tbsp reduced-fat canola oil margarine, melted
²/₃ cup ready-made apple sauce
¼ cup skim milk
²/₃ cup unsweetened cocoa powder
1½ cups self-rising flour
strawberries, to serve

CHOCOLATE ICING
1 cup confectioners' sugar, sifted
2 tbsp unsweetened cocoa powder
1–2 tbsp skim milk

PREP TIME: 20 MINUTES
COOKING TIME: 40 MINUTES
SERVINGS: 12

Preheat the oven to 350°F. Brush an 8 in kugelhopf pan with melted butter, dust lightly with flour and shake out any excess.

Whisk the eggs and sugar in a bowl for 5 minutes, or until pale and thick. Combine the margarine, apple sauce and milk in a small bowl, stirring to mix well, then fold into the egg mixture. Sift the cocoa powder and flour together into a bowl, then fold into the egg mixture.

Pour the mixture into the pan and bake for 35–40 minutes, or until a skewer inserted into the center of the cake comes out clean. Leave the cake to cool in the pan for 5 minutes, then turn out onto a wire rack to cool completely.

To make the chocolate icing, combine the confectioners' sugar and cocoa powder in a bowl, then stir in enough milk to form a thick paste. Stand the bowl over a saucepan of simmering water, stirring until the icing is smooth, then remove from the heat. Spread the icing over the cake and and arrange a few unhulled strawberries over the top. Hull and chop remainder of strawberries and serve with the cake.

This chocolate cake is best eaten on the day it is made.

nutrition per serving: Energy 234 Cal; Fat 4 g; Saturated fat 1.3 g; Protein 6 g; Carbohydrate 43.3 g; Fiber 2.3 g; Cholesterol 47 mg; Sodium 157 mg

PRUNE AND PECAN LOAF

THIS FRUIT LOAF IS DELICIOUS AND GREAT TO SERVE WHEN FRIENDS DROP BY FOR AFTERNOON TEA. IT'S A GOOD SOURCE OF FIBER AND PROVIDES SOME ANTIOXIDANTS.

canola oil spray
¼ cup light canola margarine
⅓ cup raw sugar
1 tsp natural vanilla extract
1 cup chopped pitted prunes
6½ cups pecans, chopped
1⅔ cups stoneground self-rising flour

1 tsp freshly grated nutmeg
½ cup unprocessed barley bran or oat bran

PREP TIME: 15 MINUTES
COOKING TIME: 45 MINUTES
MAKES 10–12 SLICES

Preheat the oven to 325°F. Spray a 8 x 4 in loaf pan with oil, then line the base with baking paper.

Put the margarine, sugar, vanilla, chopped prunes and pecans in a large bowl. Pour over 1 cup boiling water and stir to just melt the margarine.

Sift the flour and nutmeg into the bowl, then add the barley bran and return any husks to the bowl. Stir until well incorporated. Spoon into the prepared pan and smooth the surface.

Bake for 45 minutes, or until cooked when tested with a metal skewer. Cover with foil if the top is browning too much. Leave in the pan 10 minutes, then turn out onto a wire rack to cool. Cut into slices to serve. Serve warm or cold. Delicious toasted.

HINTS:
• Will keep refrigerated for up to 1 week, and frozen for up to 1 month.
• If you can't find barley bran in your supermarket, look for it at a health food shop.

nutrition per slice (12): Energy 210 Cal; Fat 6.2 g; Saturated fat 0.7 g; Protein 3.6 g; Carbohydrate 33.3 g; Fiber 3.8 g; Cholesterol 0 mg; Sodium 150 mg

CINNAMON, APPLE AND WALNUT CAKE

canola oil spray
1²/₃ cups stoneground self-rising flour
2 tsp ground cinnamon
½ tsp baking powder
½ cup ground almonds
¼ cup sugar
2 apples, peeled, cored and diced
½ cup chopped walnuts
2 eggs
½ cup buttermilk

½ cup unsweetened apple purée
2 tbsp canola oil

PREP TIME: 20 MINUTES
COOKING TIME: 50 MINUTES
SERVINGS: 10–12

Preheat the oven to 350°F. Spray a 9 in round cake pan with oil, then line the base with baking paper.

Sift the flour, cinnamon and baking powder into a large bowl, then return any husks to the bowl. Stir in the ground almonds and sugar, then the diced apple and chopped walnuts.

Whisk together the eggs, buttermilk, apple purée and oil in a bowl. Add to the flour mixture, then stir until combined and smooth. Spoon into the prepared pan and smooth the surface.

Bake for 50 minutes, or until cooked when tested with a metal skewer. Leave in the pan for 15 minutes, then turn out onto a wire rack to cool. Cut into wedges to serve. Delicious served warm.

HINT:
• Will keep refrigerated for up to 1 week. Freeze for up to 1 month.

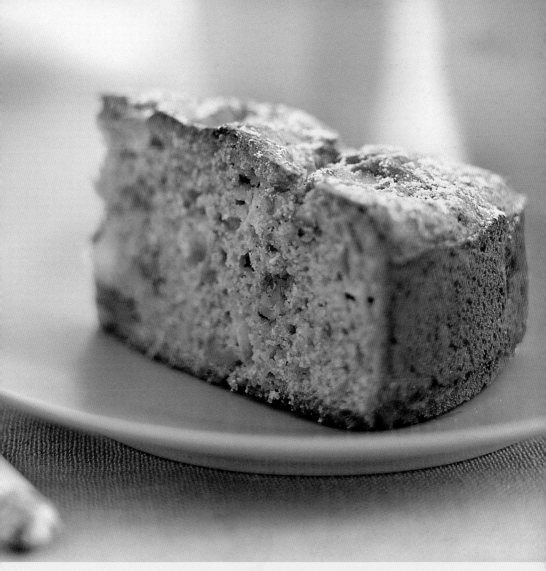

THIS SPICED APPLE CAKE IS
GREAT COMFORT FOOD, IT CAN
BE SERVED WARM OR COLD.
ENJOY IN MODERATION.

nutrition per serving: Energy 219 Cal
Fat 10.4 g
Saturated fat 1 g
Protein 5.4 g
Carbohydrate 25.1 g
Fiber 2.5 g
Cholesterol 32 mg
Sodium 194 mg

FRUIT AND TEA LOAF

THIS IS A GREAT LOW CHOLESTEROL TEA LOAF—IT DOESN'T CONTAIN ANY OIL OR BUTTER. IT'S GOOD TO SERVE ANY TIME OF DAY.

about 3 cups mixed dried fruit
¾ cup strong, hot black tea
⅔ cup lightly packed brown sugar
1 egg, lightly beaten
1 cup all-purpose flour
¾ tsp baking powder
1 tsp ground cinnamon
¼ tsp ground nutmeg
a large pinch of ground cloves

PREP TIME: 20 MINUTES + 3 HOURS SOAKING

COOKING TIME: 1 HOUR 35 MINUTES

SERVINGS: 10–12

Combine the fruit and hot tea in a large bowl, cover with plastic wrap and leave for 3 hours or overnight. Preheat the oven to 315°F. Grease a 9 x 5 in loaf pan and line the base with baking paper. Dust the sides of the tin with a little flour, shaking off any excess.

Stir the sugar and egg into the fruit mixture and combine well. Sift the flour, baking powder and spices into a bowl, then add the fruit mixture. Using a large slotted spoon, stir to combine well.

Spoon the mixture into the pan and bake for 1 hour 35 minutes, covering the top with foil if it browns too quickly. The loaf is cooked when a skewer inserted into the center of the loaf comes out clean. Cool the loaf in the pan, then turn out and serve, sliced and buttered, if desired.

The loaf will keep, wrapped in plastic wrap and stored in an airtight container in a cool place, for up to 1 week, or up to 8 weeks in the freezer.

nutrition per serving (12): Energy 199 Cal; Fat 1 g; Saturated fat 0.3 g; Protein 2.6 g; Carbohydrate 45 g; Fiber 2.9 g; Cholesterol 16 mg; Sodium 86 mg

ITALIAN DRIED FRUIT BUNS

FOR A SPECIAL TREAT, WHY NOT PUT THE KETTLE ON AND GRAB ONE OF THESE TASTY BUNS. THEY'RE LOWER IN FAT THAN SCONES AND OTHER BUNS.

¾ cup raisins

3 tsp instant dried yeast

⅓ cup sugar

3 cups flour

¼ cup unprocessed wheat or oat bran

1 tsp almond extract

1 tbsp olive oil

finely grated zest from 1 orange

¼ cup mixed peel

¼ cup pine nuts

1 egg, lightly beaten

½ cup sugar, extra

PREP TIME: 30 MINUTES + 20 MINUTES SOAKING + 2 HOURS 50 MINUTES RISING TIME

COOKING TIME: 15 MINUTES

MAKES 12

Cover the raisins with 1 cup boiling water in a small bowl and set aside for 20 minutes. Drain, reserving the liquid. Put half the liquid into a bowl, add the yeast, a pinch of the sugar and ¼ cup of the flour. Stir to combine, then leave in a draft-free place for 10 minutes, or until the yeast is foamy.

Add the remaining flour, bran, sugar and pinch of salt into the bowl of an electric mixer with a dough hook attachment and make a well in the center. Combine the remaining raisin water with the almond extract and oil, then pour it, along with the yeast mixture, into the well. Add the raisins, orange zest, mixed peel and pine nuts. With the mixer set to the lowest speed, mix until a dough forms. Increase the speed to medium and knead the dough for 5 minutes, or until it is smooth and elastic; add a little more flour if necessary. Alternatively, mix the dough by hand using a wooden spoon, then turn out onto a floured work surface and knead for 10 minutes, or until smooth and elastic.

Grease a large bowl with oil, then transfer the dough to the bowl, turning the dough to coat in the oil. Cover with plastic wrap and leave to rise in a draught-free place for 2 hours, or until the dough has doubled in size. Knock back the dough by punching it gently, then turn out onto a lightly floured work surface. Divide the dough into 12 equal portions and shape each piece into an oval. To glaze the rolls, coat them in egg, then roll them in the extra sugar to coat. Transfer the rolls to a greased baking tray and leave for 30–40 minutes, or until the rolls have risen a little (they won't quite double in size). Meanwhile, preheat the oven to 400°F. Bake the rolls for 15 minutes, or until golden, then transfer to a wire rack to cool.

nutrition per serving: Energy 266 Cal; Fat 5 g; Saturated fat 0.6 g; Protein 5.7 g; Carbohydrate 47.9 g; Fiber 3.2 g; Cholesterol 16 mg; Sodium 172 mg

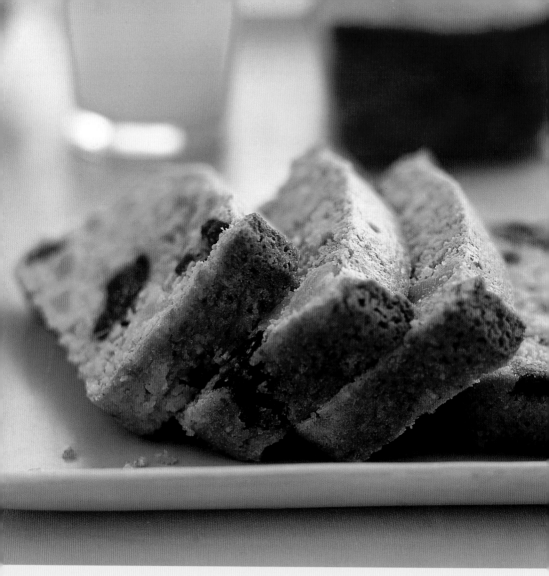

THIS DELICIOUS FRUITY BREAD
IS LOW IN FAT AND MAKES AN
EXCELLENT LIGHT MEAL OR
SNACK. ENJOY ON ITS OWN OR
WITH A LOW-FAT TOPPING.

nutrition per serving (12): Energy 180 Cal
Fat 0.9 g
Saturated fat 0.2 g
Protein 4.2 g
Carbohydrate 37.4 g
Fiber 3.9 g
Cholesterol 1 mg
Sodium 106 mg

APRICOT AND FIG BRAN BREAD

canola oil spray
1 cup unprocessed oat bran
1 cup skim or no-fat milk
½ cup dried apricots, quartered
½ cup dried figs, quartered
1 cup brown sugar
1 cup self-rising flour

1 tsp ground cinnamon

PREP TIME: 15 MINUTES + 10 MINUTES
  SOAKING TIME
COOKING TIME: 45 MINUTES
MAKES 1 LOAF (10–12 SLICES)

Preheat the oven to 350°F. Spray a 4 x 8 in loaf pan with the oil and line the base with baking paper.

Put the bran in a large bowl. Stir in the milk, dried fruit and sugar. Set aside for 10 minutes to soften the bran.

Meanwhile, sift the flour and cinnamon into a bowl. Stir the combined flour and cinnamon into the bran mixture. Pour into the prepared tin and bake for 45 minutes, or until cooked when a skewer inserted into the center of the loaf comes out clean. Cool in the pan for 10 minutes, then turn out. Cut into thick slices to serve.

HINT:
• Leftovers of this loaf are delicious when toasted. You can freeze the loaf for up to
  1 month. Use any 2–3 varieties of dried fruit or fruit medley in this recipe.

FRUIT MUFFINS

LOWER IN FAT AND CALORIES THAN MOST COMMERCIAL VARIETIES, THESE
TANGY MUFFINS ARE A GREAT SOURCE OF FIBER, POTASSIUM AND
PHOSPHORUS.

**1 cup chopped mixed dried fruit (apricots,
dates, peaches or fruit medley with peel)**
1½ cups whole-wheat self-rising flour
1 tsp baking powder
1 cup unprocessed oat bran
⅓ cup brown sugar
1¼ cups skim milk

1 egg
1 tbsp oil

PREP TIME: 15 MINUTES + 5 MINUTES
   SOAKING
COOKING TIME: 20 MINUTES
MAKES 12

Preheat the oven to moderate 350°F. Grease twelve ½ cup muffin pans. Soak the dried
fruit with ¼ cup boiling water for 5 minutes.

Sift the flour and baking powder into a large bowl, returning the husks to the bowl.
Stir in the oat bran and sugar and make a well in the center.

Combine the milk, egg and oil in a jug. Add the soaked fruit and milk mixture all at once to
the dry ingredients. Fold in gently using a metal spoon, until just combined—do not overmix.

Divide the mixture evenly among the muffin pans. Bake for 20 minutes, or until the
muffins are risen and golden, and a skewer inserted into the center comes out clean.
Cool for a few minutes in the tin, then turn out onto a wire rack. Serve warm or at
room temperature.

nutrition per muffin: Energy 192 Cal; Fat 3.3 g; Saturated fat 0.5 g; Protein 6.3 g; Carbohydrate 32.2
g; Fiber 5.1 g; Cholesterol 16 mg; Sodium 204 mg

APPLE AND PEACH MUFFINS

THESE MUFFINS ARE QUICK AND EASY TO MAKE AS THE INGREDIENTS ARE
ONLY LIGHTLY MIXED INSTEAD OF BEATEN SMOOTH. YOU CAN QUICKLY WHIP
UP A BATCH FOR A SPECIAL BREAKFAST OR AN AFTERNOON TREAT.

canola oil spray
1 cup stoneground self-rising flour
½ cup whole-wheat stoneground self-rising flour
1½ tsp ground cinnamon
½ tsp baking powder
½ cup rolled barley or oats
⅓ cup brown sugar
1 cup dried peaches, chopped
1 large green apple, peeled, cored and finely chopped

1 egg
1 cup skim milk
¼ cup reduced-fat canola margarine, just melted

PREP TIME: 20 MINUTES
COOKING TIME: 25 MINUTES
MAKES 12

Preheat the oven to 325°F. Spray muffin pan with oil.

Sift the flours, cinnamon and baking powder into a large bowl, then return any husks to the bowl. Stir in the rolled barley, brown sugar, chopped peaches and chopped apple. Make a well in the center.

Whisk together the egg, milk and melted margarine and stir into the flour mixture until just combined. Do not overmix. Spoon evenly into the muffin pan.

Bake for 20–25 minutes, or until firm to touch and golden brown. Leave in the pan for 5 minutes, then turn out onto a wire rack to cool. Delicious served warm or cold.

HINTS:
• Will keep refrigerated for up to 5 days or frozen for up to 1 month.
• To lower the calories and GI slightly, you can use half sucralose and half sugar instead of sugar only, but the end result will not be quite so light and fluffy.

nutrition per muffin: Energy 168 Cal; Fat 3.4 g; Saturated fat 1.1 g; Protein 4.5 g; Carbohydrate 29 g; Fiber 3.2 g; Cholesterol 16 mg; Sodium 188 mg

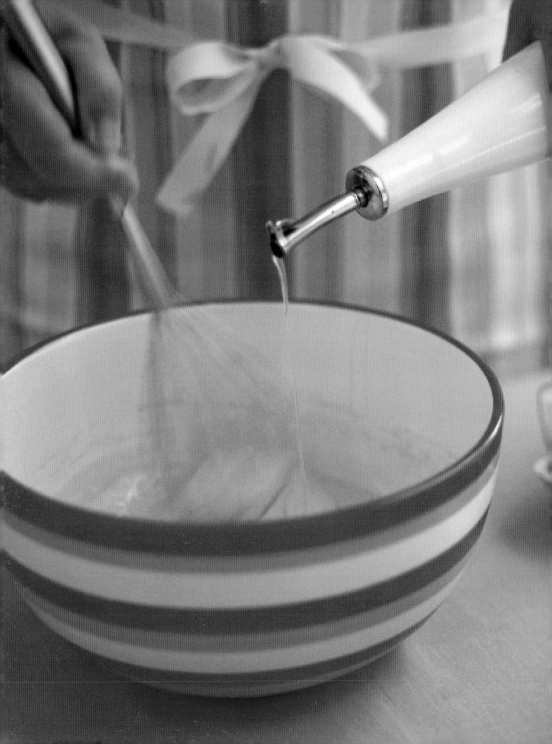

Contact information

USA
American Heart Association
727 Greenville Avenue
Dallas, Texas 75231
Phone: 1 800 242 8721
Web: www.americanheart.org

CANADA
Heart and Stroke Foundation of Canada
222 Queen St, Suite 1402
Ottawa, ON K1P 5V9
Phone: 613 569 4361
Web: www.heartandstroke.ca

UNITED KINGDOM
The British Heart Foundation
14 Fitzhardinge St
London W1H D6H
Phone: 020 7935 0185
Web: www.bhf.org.uk

AUSTRALIA
National Heart Foundation of Australia
Phone: 02 6232 3800
Heart line: 1300 36 27 87
Web: www.heartfoundation.com.au

Heart Research Institute
145–147 Missenden Road
Camperdown NSW 2050
Phone: 02 8208 8900
Web: www.hri.org.au

NEW ZEALAND
National Heart Foundation of New Zealand
9 Kalmia St
Ellerslie, Auckland 1130
Phone: 09 571 9191
Web: www.nhf.org.nz

INDEX